The Keto Diet Culinary Bo

150+ Culinary Ideas of 2021 for a Healthy and
(with pictures)

By

Gianna Carter

Author : Gianna Carter

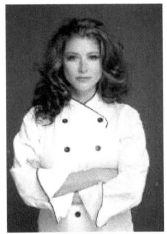

Gianna Carter is a nutritionist who specializes in the ketogenic diet and exercise physiology in 2015. He struggled with his health and her weight in childhood which led to her becoming such a passionate nutrition expert. "My goal is to help transform people lives and start living again!" Jamie spends most of his time with clients around the world via online coaching with amazing and measurable results. She specializes in helping autoimmune diseases, diabetes (type 1 and type 2), heart disease, cholesterol problems, alopecia, cancer, epilepsy, seizures, depression and anxiety. You'd be amazed at the number of people who stop taking drugs with her guidance. She helped thousands of clients over the past 5 years.

She is also an author of over 30 books from the 2 massive series: "Air Fryer Boot Camp" & "The Rules of Ketogenic Life", currently available!

Table of Contents

The 15-Day Keto Fasting Cookbook

Keto Dessert & Chaffle Cookbook 2021 with Pictures

The Complete Ketogenic Guidebook for Women Over 50

Easy Anti-inflammatory Recipes to Lose Belly Fat, Boost your Metabolism, and increase your energy above the age of 50

By
Gianna Carter

Table of contents

Introduction

A Keto diet is one that is very low in carbohydrates but rich in fats and is normal on protein. Through the years, the Keto diet has been used to treat a variety of diseases that people have learned to face. This includes: rectifying weight gain as well as managing or treating diseases of human beings like treating epilepsy in youngsters. The Keto diet enables the human body to use its fats instead of consuming its carbohydrates. Typically, the body's carbohydrates, which are present in the foods you eat, are transformed into glucose. Glucose is a consequence of the body burning off its carbohydrates which are typically distributed throughout the body. A dietary strategy and a balanced lifestyle are, thus, an important necessity for all the citizens who choose to prevent early mortality. Health problems are widely prevalent in women over the age of 50 since they suffer from normal bodily adjustments related to menopause.

Osteoporosis, hypertension, high blood pressure, overweight, and inflammation are popular among women of this category. An effective metabolism is a secret to good health! The level of metabolism does not stay the same, though! As an individual age, the body naturally moves through a slow metabolic phase. This phase of aging speeds up as we eat unhealthy food and live an unhealthy lifestyle, resulting in a variety of metabolic disorders and other associated diseases. It's a popular myth that you'll be consuming bland and fatty food while you're on a ketogenic diet. Although basic foods are a necessity, there are so many ways to bring the spice back into your diet.

Doing keto doesn't just include consuming any type of fat or having ice cream on the mouth. Instead, it's about choosing products that are high in healthy fats and poor in carbohydrates cautiously. If you aren't sure where to go, don't be afraid. Some really good, fantastic keto meals are out there promising to be eaten.

Chapter 1: Introduction to Ketogenic Diet

A ketogenic diet is widely known as a diet which is low in carbs and in which the human body generates ketones to be processed as energy in the liver. Several different names are related to a keto diet, lower-carb diet, lower-carb high fat (LCHF), etc. Patterns of diet come and go, and it seems like the formula mostly includes a low-carb plan. At the top of the chart right now is the ketogenic diet. The keto diet, also referred to as the ketogenic diet, relies on having more of the calories from protein and a few from fat while eliminating carbohydrates dramatically.

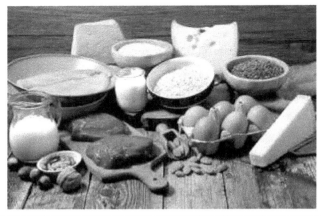

1.1 How Does The Ketogenic Diet Work?

A high fat, medium protein, low carbohydrate diet plan, which varies from standard, balanced eating recommendations, is the ketogenic diet. Many foods abundant in nutrients, including vegetables, fruits, whole grains, milk products, are sources of carbohydrates. Carbs from both types are highly constrained on a keto diet. Keto dieters, therefore, do not eat bread, grains, or cereals with the intention of holding carbs below 50 g a day. And since them, too, contain carbohydrates, even fruits and vegetables are restricted. The keto diet involves making drastic changes about how they normally consume for most individuals.

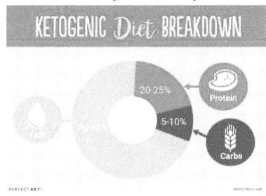

What is Ketosis?

Ketosis is a metabolic condition where the body utilizes fat and ketones as the main source of fuel instead of glucose (sugar).

A critical part of beginning a keto diet is knowing how Ketosis works. Ketosis, irrespective of the number of carbohydrates you consume, is a phase that the body goes through on a daily basis. This is because if sugar is not readily accessible, this method provides humans energy from ketones.

HOW TO GET INTO KETOSIS

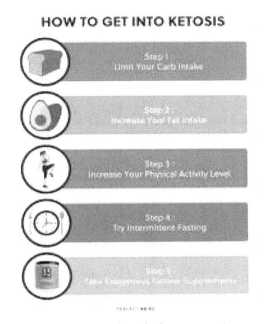

The body tends to raise its ketone levels if the requirement for energy grows, and carbohydrates are not sufficient to satisfy the need. If a more extended period of time (i.e., more than three days) is limited to carbohydrates, the body can raise ketone levels much more. These deeper ketosis rates produce several favorable benefits in the body, results that are achieved when adopting the ketogenic diet is the best and healthiest manner practicable.

Most individuals, however, seldom get Ketosis and never feel its advantages because the body tends to use sugar as its main source of power, even if the diet provides plenty of carbohydrates and protein.

How does Ketosis happen?

The body would turn any of its accumulated fat into extremely effective energy molecules called ketones while the body has no access to healthy food, like while you are resting, exercising, or adopting a ketogenic diet. (We should credit our body's capacity to alter metabolic processes for that.) After the body breaks down fat into glycerol and fatty acids, such ketones are synthesized.

While in certain cells in the body, fatty acids and glycerol may be directly converted into food, brain cells do not use them as energy at all. This really is because they are so gradually processed into energy to help the brain work.

That's why sugar appears to be the brain's primary source of fuel. Interestingly, this also enables one to realize that we make ketones. Thus providing an alternate source of energy, because we do not eat sufficient calories, our brain will be incredibly susceptible. Our muscles will be quickly broken down and transformed into glucose to support our brains that are sugar-hungry before we have enough power left to find food. The human species would most definitely be endangered without ketones.

1.2 Types of Ketogenic Diet

There are a variety of aspects in which ketosis can be induced, and so there are a number of diverse ketogenic diet variations.

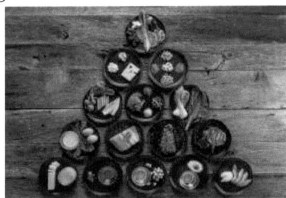

Keto Diet Standard (SKD)

This is a really low carb diet, a medium protein diet yet high fat. Usually, it comprises 70 to 75% fat, 20% protein, and only 5 to 10% carbohydrates.

A traditional standard ketogenic diet, in terms of grams per day, will be:

- Carbohydrate between 20-50g
- Around 40-60g of protein
- No limit specified for fat

The bulk of calories should be given by fat in the diet for this to be a keto diet. As energy needs might differ greatly among individuals, no limit is set. A large number of vegetables, especially non-starchy veggies, should be included in ketogenic diets, as they are very low in carbs.

In order to help people reduce weight, increase blood glucose regulation and improve cardiac health, standardized ketogenic diets have repeatedly demonstrated success.

Very-low-carb diet ketogenic (VLCKD)

Very-low-carb is a traditional ketogenic diet, and so a VLCKD would normally correspond to a traditional ketogenic diet.

Ketogenic Diet Well Formulated (WFKD)

The word 'Well Formulated Keto Diet' derives from one of the main ketogenic diet experts, Steve Phinney.

As a traditional ketogenic diet, the WFKD maintains a similar blueprint. Well-developed ensures that weight, protein & carbohydrate macronutrients align with the ratios of the traditional ketogenic diet and thus have the greatest likelihood of ketosis happening.

Ketogenic Diet MCT

This fits the description of the traditional ketogenic diet but insists on providing more of the diet's fat content through the use of medium-chain triglycerides (MCTs). MCTs are present in coconut oil and are accessible in the liquid state of MCT oil and MCT dispersant.

To treat epilepsy, MCT ketogenic diets are being used since the idea is that MCTs enable individuals to absorb more carbohydrates and protein, thus sustaining ketosis. That's because multiple ketones per gram of fat are produced by MCTs than the long-chain triglycerides found in natural dietary fat. There is a dearth of research, though, exploring whether MCTs have greater advantages on weight loss and blood sugar.

Ketogenic diet Calorie-restricted

Unless calories are reduced to a fixed number, a calorie-restricted ketogenic diet is identical to a normal ketogenic diet.

Research indicates that, whether calorie consumption is reduced or not, ketogenic diets seem to be effective. This is because it helps to avoid over-eating of itself from the nutritious impact of eating fat and staying in ketosis.

The Ketogenic Cyclical Diet (CKD)

There are days on which more carbohydrates are ingested, like five ketogenic days accompanied by two high carbohydrate days, in the CKD diet, frequently recognized as carb back loading.

The diet is meant for athletes who can regenerate glycogen drained from muscles during exercises using the high carbohydrate days.

Ketogenic Diet Targeted (TKD)

Even though carbs are eaten around exercise hours, the TKD is equivalent to a typical ketogenic diet. It is a combination between a regular ketogenic diet as well as a cyclical ketogenic diet that requires every day you work out to eat carbohydrates.

It is focused on the assumption that carbohydrates eaten before or during a physical effort can be absorbed even more effectively, while the need for energy from the muscles rises while we are engaged.

Ketogenic Diet of High Protein

With a proportion of 35 percent protein, 60 percent fat, and 5 percent carbohydrates, this diet contains more protein than a regular keto diet.

For people who need to lose weight, a study shows that a high-protein keto is beneficial for weight loss. Like in other types of the ketogenic diet, if practiced for several years, there is an absence of research on which there are any health risks.

1.3 Benefits of Ketogenic Diet

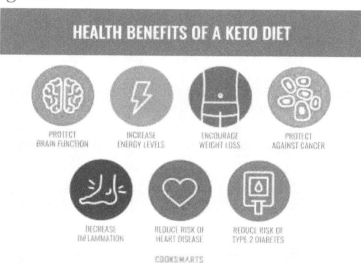

A keto diet has many advantages, including:

Weight Reduction

A person's keto diet will help them lose weight. The keto diet help encourages weight loss in many aspects, particularly metabolism boosting and appetite reduction. Ketogenic diets comprise foods that load up an individual and can minimize hormones that trigger appetite. For these factors, it may suppress appetite and encourage weight loss by adopting a keto diet.

Helps improve acne

In certain persons, acne has many common reasons and can have associations with diet and blood sugar. Consuming a diet rich in highly processed carbs can change the equivalence of intestinal bacteria and cause major rises and declines in blood sugar, both of which would negatively impact the health of the skin.

It can decrease the risk of certain cancers.

The implications of the ketogenic diet have been studied by experts to potentially avoid or even cure some cancers. One research showed that in patients with some cancers, a ketogenic diet could be a healthy and appropriate complementary medication to be used in addition to chemotherapy and radiation therapy. This is because, in cancer cells, it might cause greater oxidative stress than in regular cells, allowing them to die.

It can safeguard brain function.

Some research indicates that neuroprotective advantages are offered by the ketones developed during the ketogenic diet that indicates they can reinforce and defend the brain and nerve cells.

A ketogenic diet might help a person resist or maintain problems such as Alzheimer's disease for this purpose.

Lessens seizures potentially

In a ketogenic diet, the proportion of fat, protein, and carbohydrates changes the way the body utilizes energy, results in ketosis. Ketosis is a biochemical mechanism in which ketone bodies are being used by the body for energy.

The Epilepsy Foundation indicates that ketosis in people with epilepsy, particularly those who have not adapted to other types of treatment, might decrease seizures. More study is required on how efficient this is, as it seems to have the greatest influence on children who have generalized seizures.

Improves the effects of PCOS

Polycystic ovary syndrome (PCOS) may contribute to surplus male hormones, ovulatory instability, and polycystic ovaries as a hormonal syndrome. In individuals with PCOS, a high-carbohydrate diet can trigger negative impacts, like skin problems as well as excess weight.

The researchers observed that many markers of PCOS are strengthened by a ketogenic diet, including:

- Loss in weight
- Balance of hormones
- Ratios of follicle-stimulating hormone (LH) and luteinizing hormone (LH) (FSH)
- Insulin fasting levels

A different research analysis showed that for people with hormonal conditions, like PCOS and type 2 diabetes, a keto diet has positive benefits. They also cautioned, though, that the findings were too diverse to prescribe a keto diet as a specific PCOS treatment.

Chapter 2: Easy ketogenic Low Carb Recipes

It may be challenging to adopt different diets: all the foods to quit, to consume more, to purchase new products. It's enough to make bonkers for everyone. But the ketogenic, or "keto," diet, as well as its keto meals, are one type of eating that has been gathering traction lately.

Doing keto doesn't only involve eating some sort of fat or putting ice cream on your mouth. Rather, it's about picking items that are rich in good fats and low in carbohydrates carefully. If you aren't sure where to start, don't be scared. Some very healthy, excellent keto meals are out there appealing to be consumed.

2.1 Keto Breakfast Recipes

1. HIGH PROTEIN COTTAGE CHEESE OMELET

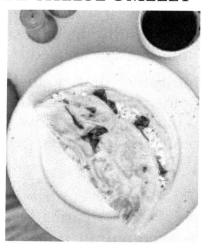

Serving: 1

Preparation time: 5 minutes

Nutritional Values: 250kcal Calories | 18g Fat | 4 g Carbs | 18.7g Proteins

Ingredients

- 2 eggs - large
- 1 tbsp. of whole milk or 2% milk
- Kosher salt about 1/8 tsp.
- Pinch of black pepper, freshly ground,
- 1/2 tbsp. of butter - unsalted
- 1 cup spinach (about 1 ounce)
- Cottage cheese 3 tbsp.

Directions

1. In a moderate pan, put the eggs, milk, salt, & pepper and stir until the whites & yolks are thoroughly combined, and the eggs are a little viscous.

2. In an 8-inch non - stick roasting pan over medium heat, add the butter. Flip the pan until the butter covers the bottom equally. Include the spinach and simmer for around 30 seconds before it is ripened. Put the eggs in and turn the pan directly so that the eggs cover the whole bottom.

3. To softly pull and move the cooked eggs from the sides into the middle of the pan, use either a silicone or rubber spatula, leaving room for the raw eggs and creating waves in the omelet. Rig a spatula underneath the edges to enable raw eggs to run beneath the cooked part, holding and swiveling the pan. Cook for around 2 minutes until the sides are settled, and the middle is moist but no longer soft or gooey.

4. Let the pan away from the heat. Whisk over half the eggs with the cottage cheese. Cover the egg carefully over the filling using a spatula. On a plate, transfer the omelet.

2. DEVILED EGGS

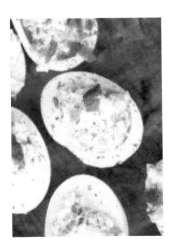

Serving: 4-6

Preparation time: 15-20 minutes

Nutritional values: 280kcal Calories | 23g Fat | 3.4g Carbs | 15g Proteins

Ingredients

- 12 eggs - large
- 8 oz. of full-fat cream cheese, warmed for 1 hour or more at room temperature,
- Kosher salt about 1/2 teaspoon
- 1 shred of black pepper
- 2 tablespoons of all the bagel seasoning

Directions

1. A dozen eggs become hardboiled according to your chosen method. (The most critical part is to layer with ice water, raise to a boil, then lift from the heat and leave for 8 to 10 minutes to remain.) In an ice bucket, soak and chill the eggs. And peel them.

2. Cut the eggs laterally in half and use a tiny spoon to pick the yolks out and put them in a dish.

3. Take the cream cheese and transfer it to the yolks into rough parts. Use a hand beater or stick mixer to mix until smooth and blended, starting at lower speeds and then at high speed. Bang in the pepper and salt. Uh, taste. If needed, tweak the seasonings.

4. Load the egg whites with the yolk mixture using a spoon or piping bag. (It would be stiff; to soften it any further if possible, microwave it in very fast bursts of 2 to 3 seconds.)

5. With the all-bagel seasoning, dust the tops of the loaded eggs appropriately. In two hours, serve.

3. 90 SECOND KETO BREAD

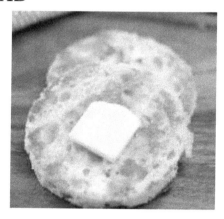

Serving: 1

Preparation time: 90 seconds

Nutritional values: 99kcal Calories | 8.5g Fat | 2g Carbs | 3.9g Proteins

Instructions

- 1 egg - large
- 1 spoonful of milk
- Olive oil about 1 tablespoon
- 1 tablespoon flour of coconut
- 1 tablespoon flour of almonds or hazelnuts

- 1/4 tsp. powder for baking
- Pinch of salt

Add-ins optional:

- 1/4 cup of grated cheese
- 1 tbsp. scallions or herbs chopped

Directions

1. In a small cup, mix together the egg, milk, oil, coconut flour, almond flour, baking powder, and salt. If using, incorporate cheese and scallions or herbs and mix to blend.

2. To induce any air bubbles to lift and burst, pour into a wide microwave-safe mug and strike the bottom tightly on the counter multiple times. Reheat for 1 minute, 30 seconds, on maximum.

3. On a chopping board, transpose the mug and enable the bread to drop out. Slice into 1/2-inch-thick strips crosswise. For the toast, heat a teaspoon of oil across moderate flame in a small pan until it glistens. Add the strips and toast, around 30 seconds on either side, before golden-brown.

4. KETO FRITTATA

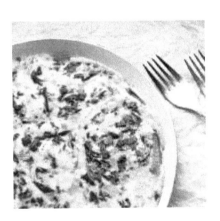

Serving: 4-6

Preparation time: 25 minutes

Nutritional values: 155kcal Calories | 8.9g Fat | 11.4g Carbs | 7.9g Proteins

Instructions

- 6 large eggs, sufficient for the ingredients to fill
- Heavy cream 1/4 cup
- 1 tsp. of kosher salt, split-up
- 4 thick-cut bacon (8 oz.) pieces, diced (optional)

- 2 tiny, stripped, and finely diced Yukon gold potatoes
- 1/4 tsp. of black pepper, freshly ground
- 2 cups of spinach (2 ounces)
- Garlic 2 cloves, chopped.
- 2 tsp. of fresh leaves of thyme
- 1 cup of Gruyere, Fontina, or Cheddar crushed cheese

Directions

1. Preheat oven. In the center of the oven, position a brace and warm it to 400 °F.

2. Stir together the cream and eggs. In a medium bowl, stir together the eggs, whipping cream, and 1/2 teaspoon salt; hold.

3. Just prepare the bacon. Put the bacon in a non - stick 10-12-inch cold cooking pan or cast-iron skillet, and keep the heat to moderate. Cook the bacon until translucent, stirring regularly, for 8 to 10 minutes. Move the bacon to a paper towel-lined dish with a slotted spoon and skim off all but 2 tbsp. of the fat. (If the bacon is excluded, heat the pan with 2 tablespoons of oil, then finish incorporating the potatoes).

4. Simmer the potatoes in the fat of the bacon. Mix the potatoes and spray with the pepper and the remaining 1/2 teaspoon salt. Switch the pan to a moderate flame. Heat, stirring regularly, for 4 to 6 minutes, until soft and golden brown.

5. Crumble the spinach with thyme & garlic. Put the spinach, garlic, and thyme in the pan and cook, mixing, for 30 seconds to 1 minute, or until the spinach is wilted. Transfer the bacon again to the skillet and swirl to spread uniformly.

6. Add some cheese. Scattered the vegetables, compressed with a spatula, into an even layer. Over the top, spread the cheese and let it only begin to melt.

7. In the pan, add the egg mixture. Place over the vegetables and cheese with the egg mixture. To be sure that the eggs settle equally over all the vegetables, rotate the skillet. Wait for a minute or two before you observe the eggs starting to set at the ends of the pan.

8. Around 8 to 10 minutes, oven the frittata. Bake for 8 to 10 minutes unless the eggs are ready. Cut a tiny slit in the middle of the frittata to test. Bake for a few more minutes if uncooked eggs run into the cut; if the eggs are fixed, take the frittata out of the oven. At the end of cooking, hold the frittata underneath the broiler for a couple of minutes for a crisped, charred layer.

9. For 5 minutes, chill in the skillet, then cut into slices and serve.

5. CHEESE, HAM, AND EGG WRAPS

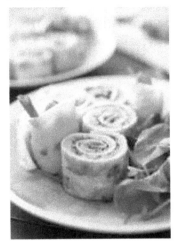

Serving: 4

Preparation time: 15-20 minutes

Nutritional values: 371kcal calories | 27g Fat | %g Carbs | 27g Proteins

Ingredients

- 8 eggs - large
- 4 tsp. of Water
- 2 tsp. of all-purpose or cornstarch flour
- Half a teaspoon of fine salt
- 4 tsp. of coconut or vegetable oil
- 1 1/3 cups of Swiss grated cheese
- 4 ounces of ham extremely thinly sliced
- 1 1/3 cups of watercress loosely wrapped

Directions

1. In a wide bowl, put the eggs, water, flour or cornflour, and salt, and stir until the starch or cornflour is fully dissolved.

2. In a 12-inch non - stick saucepan, heat 1 tsp. Of oil unless glinting, over moderate flame. To cover the surface with the oil, move the pan. To brush the bottom part in a thin coating, incorporate 1/2 cup of the egg mixture and stir. Cook for 3 to 6 minutes before the wrapping is fully set on the sides and on the surface (the top may be a little damp but should be apparently set).

3. Soften the sides of the wrap using a wide spatula and move it under the wrap, ensuring that it will slide across the pan quickly. With the spatula, turn the wrap. Slather 1/3 cup of cheese instantly over the wrap and simmer

for around 1 minute before the second side is ready. Drop it onto a chopping board or work surface (the cheese may not be completely melted yet). Put a single coat of ham over the egg when it is still hot. Put 1/3 of a cup of watercress in the middle of the wrap. Firmly roll it up.

4. Repeat the leftover wraps by cooking and filling them. Slice each wrap crosswise into 6 (1-inch) bits using a steak knife.

6. BACON GRUYERE EGG BITES

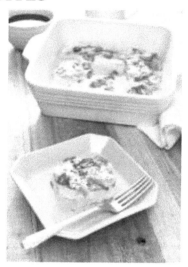

Serving: 9

Preparation time: 10-20 minutes

Nutritional values: 208kcal Calories | 18g Fat | 1g Carbs | 11g Proteins

Ingredients

- Fat or butter of bacon, to coat the pan
- 9 large eggs
- 3/4 cup Gruyere cheese grated (2 1/4 oz.)
- 1/3 cup (about 2 1/2 oz.) cream cheese
- Kosher salt about 1/2 teaspoon
- 6 pieces of thick-cut, cooked, and imploded bacon

Directions

1. In the center of the oven, place a rack and warm it to 350°F. Graciously cover an 8x8-inch (broiler-safe if you like a crisped top) cooking dish with bacon fat or butter.

2. Put the eggs, Gruyere, cream cheese, and salt in a mixer and combine for around 1 minute, at moderate speed, until quite smooth. Drop it into the pan for baking. Slather bacon with it. With aluminum foil, cover firmly.

3. Take the oven rack out from the oven midway. Upon on the oven rack, put a roasting tray. Put in 6 extremely hot tap water pots. Place the baking dish in the hot skillet with the eggs. Bake until the center is just ready, 55 minutes to 1 hour.

4. Pull the roasting pan from the oven cautiously. Remove the roasting pan from the baking dish and unfold it. (For a browned surface: Heat the oven to sauté. Sauté 4 to 5 minutes before the top is golden-brown.) Slice and serve into 9 squares.

7. RADISH TURNIP AND FRIED EGGS HASH WITH GREEN GARLIC

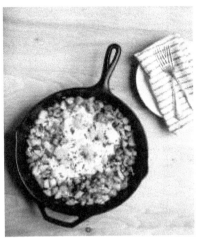

Serving: 2

Preparation time: 10-12 minutes

Nutritional values: 392kcal calories | 34g Fat | 10g Carbs | 13g Proteins

Ingredients

- 2 to 3 tiny turnips (approximately 1 1/2 cups cubed) clipped, peeled, and sliced into 3/4-inch cubes
- 4 to 5 tiny, rinsed and clipped radishes, and sliced into 3/4-inch cubes (approximately 1 1/2 cubed cups)
- Crushed Salt of the Sea
- Pepper freshly crushed
- 2 tbsp. of grapeseed oil, or other heat-tolerant, neutral oil
- 1 green garlic stalk, clipped and diced (just white and light green parts)
- 2 spoonful's of unsalted butter
- Four eggs
- 1 tablespoon parsley chopped

Directions

1. Place the water in a wide skillet and raise it to a boil. Stir in 2 teaspoons of sea salt. Transfer to a bowl with a slotted spoon, skim off any extra water and set it aside. Simmer turnip cubes only until moist, 3 to 4 minutes. Next, quickly boil the radishes for 30 to 60 seconds; scrape with a slotted spoon in a pan, skim off any extra water, and set it aside.

2. Place a sauté pan of cast iron over moderate flame. Include the grapeseed oil and add the turnips & radishes when warm, and pinch the sea salt and pepper with each one. Cook for 8 minutes or until golden-brown, flipping vegetables just once or twice. Switch the heat to medium, bring in the green garlic and simmer for a minute or so. Place the vegetables to the edges, melt the butter in the center of the pan, and add the eggs. Cook unearthed for 4 to 6 minutes for over-easy eggs; close pan for 3 minutes for over-medium eggs, then unfold and continue to cook only until whites are ready, 2 to 3 minutes further. To taste, finish with chopped parsley and sea salt and pepper. Instantly serve.

8. CAULIFLOWER RICE BURRITO BOWLS

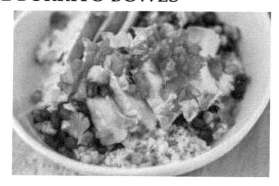

Serving: 4

Preparation time: 20-25 minutes

Nutritional values: 374kcal Calories | 15g Fat | 46g Carbs | 21g Protein

Ingredients

- 1 (15-ounce) canned washed and cleaned black beans.
- 1 cup of corn kernels - frozen
- 2 spoonful's of water
- Chili powder about 1/2 teaspoon
- 1/2 teaspoon of cumin powder
- 3/4 teaspoon of kosher salt, distributed
- 1 tablespoon of olive oil

- One cauliflower of a medium head (just around 1 1/2 lbs.), riced (or one 16oz sack riced cauliflower)
- 1/3 cup of fresh cilantro minced, distributed
- 1/4 cup of lime juice, freshly extracted (from 2 to 3 lemons)
- 1 cup roasted chicken chopped or shredded (optional), warmed if necessary
- 1 cup of gallo pico de or salsa
- One large, drained, pitted, and diced avocado

Directions

1. In a small pan, put the beans, corn, water, chili powder, cumin, and 1/4 tsp. over moderate flame. Cook for 3 to 5 minutes, mixing periodically until hot. Distance yourself from the steam.

2. In the meantime, over a moderate flame, heat the oil in a wide, large skillet until it shimmers. Transfer the cauliflower and the residual 1/2 teaspoon salt to the mixture. Process until the cauliflower is cooked through though soft, 3 to 5 minutes, mixing periodically. Remove from the heat. Transfer the cilantro and lime juice to 1/4 cup and mix to blend.

3. Divide into four bowls the riced cauliflower. Cover with the mixture of bean and corn, chicken if used, pico de gallo or salsa, and pieces of avocado. Slather with the cilantro that persists and serve hot.

9. KETO LOAF

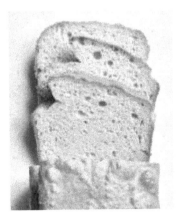

Serving: 1

Preparation time: 10-12 minutes

Nutritional values: 239kcal Calories | 22g Fat | 4g carbs | 8g Proteins

Ingredients

- Two cups of fine powdered almond flour, especially brands like King Arthur
- 1 tsp. powder for baking
- 1/2 tsp. of gum xanthan

- Kosher salt about 1\2 tsp.
- 7 eggs - large
- 8 tbsp. (1 stick) of melted and chilled unsalted butter
- 2 tbsp. of concentrated, processed, and chilled coconut oil

Directions

1. In the center of the oven, place a rack and warm it to 351°F. Cover the bottom part of a parchment paper 9x5-inch metallic loaf pan, having the surplus spill around the long sides to create a loop. Just set aside.

2. In a wide dish, mix together the flour of almond, powder for baking, xanthan gum, as well as salt. Just placed back.

3. Put the eggs in a bowl equipped with the whisk extension of a stand blender. Beat at moderate pressure until soft and drippy. Lower the level to moderate, incorporate the butter and oil of coconut gradually, and whisk unless well mixed. Lessen the intensity to medium, incorporate the mixture of almond flour gradually, and mix unless mixed. Rise the pace to moderate and beat for around 1 minute before the mixture thickens.

4. Pour and scrape the top into the primed pan. Bake for 45 to 55 minutes unless a knife placed in the middle comes out clean. Let it cool for around ten minutes in the pan. Take the loaf over the skillet, grab the parchment paper, and shift it to a cutting board. Cool it down completely until slicing.

10. BREAKFAST SALAD

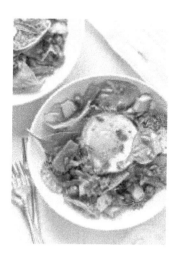

Serving: 4

Preparation time: 10 minutes

Nutritional values: 425kcal Calories | 34g Fat | 16g Carbs | 17g Proteins

Ingredients

- Spinach 8 Oz (about 6 packed cups)

- 1/2 a cup of blueberries
- 1 medium-sized avocado, chopped
- 1/3 cup red roasted quinoa
- 1/4 cup of pumpkin seeds - toasted
- Bacon - 6 strips
- 4 eggs of large size
- 1/4 cup of apple cider vinegar
- 2 tsp. of honey
- Kosher salt about 1\2 tsp.

Directions

1. In a large bowl, add the spinach, avocado, berries, pumpkin seeds, and quinoa and toss them to mix. Distribute the salad into deep plates or pots.

2. Put the bacon over moderate heat in a large cast-iron pan. Cook until the fat has dried out and the bacon is crunchy, tossing halfway around for a total of around 10 minutes. Shift the bacon to a tray that is lined with paper towels. Cut the bacon into little crumbles until it is cold.

3. Lower the heat and fry the eggs to the perfect braising in the dried bacon fat. Keep the pan away from the heat. Place the toppled bacon and an egg on top of each salad.

4. Upon emulsification, mix the vinegar, honey, and salt into the residual bacon fat in the dish. Sprinkle over the salad with the warm dressing and serve promptly.

2.2 Keto Lunch & Dinner Recipes

1. CAULIFLOWER FRIED RICE

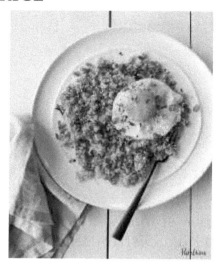

Serving: 4

Preparation time: 20- 25 minutes

Nutritional values: 108kcal Calories | 1g Fat | 21g Carbs | 7g Proteins

Ingredients

For Fried Rice

- 1 cauliflower head, sliced into cloves
- Balanced Oil 2 tbsp. (such as vegetable, coconut, or peanut)
- 1 bunch of finely sliced scallions
- 3 cloves of garlic, chopped
- 1 tbsp. natural ginger diced
- 2 peeled and finely chopped carrots
- 2 stalks of celery, chopped
- 1 bell pepper, red, chopped
- 1 cup of peas - frozen
- 2 tbsp. vinegar for rice
- 3 spoonful's of soy sauce
- Sriracha 2 tsp., or enough to taste

For Garnishing

- Balanced oil about 1tbsp. (such as vegetable, coconut, or peanut)
- Four eggs

- Salt and black pepper finely processed
- 4 tbsp. of fresh cilantro, diced
- 4 tbsp. of scallions thinly diced
- 4 tsp. of seeds of sesame

Directions

1. **For Fried Rice:** Pump the cauliflower in the mixing bowl for 2 or 3 minutes before the mishmash resembles rice. Just set aside.

2. Heat oil over a moderate flame in a wide skillet. Include the scallions, garlic, and ginger and mix for around 1 minute, unless aromatic.

3. Incorporate the carrots, celery & red bell pepper, and braise for 9 to 11 minutes until the veggies are soft.

4. Add the cauliflower rice, then stir-fry for another 3 to 5 minutes, once it starts to turn golden. To blend, mix in the frozen peas and toss properly.

5. To combine, incorporate rice vinegar, Sriracha, and soy sauce & swirl. Just set aside.

6. **For Garnishing:** Add the oil in a large skillet over moderate to high flame. Crack the eggs straight into the skillet and stir for 3 to 4 minutes before the whites are assertive, but the yolks are still watery. With pepper and salt, sprinkle each one.

7. Distribute the cauliflower rice into four dishes to serving and serve each one with a fried egg. Sprinkle with 1 tablespoon of cilantro, 1 tablespoon of scallions, and 1 teaspoon of sesame seeds on each dish. Instantly serve then.

2. LOW CARB THAI CURRY SOUP

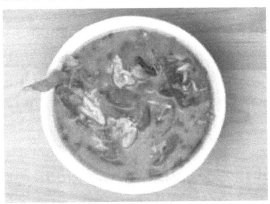

Serving: 6

Preparation time: 22 minutes

Nutritional values: 324kcal Calories | 27g Fat | 7g Carbs | 15g Proteins

Ingredients

- 4 Leg pieces of boneless skinless chicken,
- 14.5 ounces (411.07 g) full-fat coconut milk
- 2 tsp. of Thai paste of yellow curry
- 2 tsp. of fish sauce
- Three tsp. of Soy Sauce
- 1 tsp. of Agave or honey nectar
- 2 green Scallions minced
- Garlic 4 cloves, minced
- 2 inch (2 inches) coarsely chopped diced ginger

Veggies to add in soup

- One Can of Straw Mushrooms (optional)
- 74.5 g (1/2 cup) of Cherry Tomatoes, half-sliced
- Cilantro, 1/4 cup (4 g), diced
- 3 green Scallions diced
- 1 lime, juiced

Directions

For the Instant Pot

1. Put the essential soup components and lock in an Instant Pot.
2. Process it under heat for 12 minutes by using the SOUP key. The soup button avoids it from boiling and extracting the coconut milk.
3. Discharge the pressure immediately and detach and cut the chicken. Place it in the broth again.
4. Transfer the warm broth to the vegetables. In the hot broth, you want to bring them a little scorching but not to mold them though you can actually taste the flavor of the vegetables and herbs.

For the Slow Cooker

1. In a slow cooker, put the essential soup ingredients and steam for 8 hours on lower or 4 hours on average.
2. Over the last half-hour, place in vegetables and herbs. In the hot broth, you want to bring them a little scorching but not to mold them though you can actually taste the flavor of the vegetables and herbs.

3. Remove the chicken and cut it. Place it in the broth again.

- It's actually cheaper to purchase Thai Yellow Curry Paste than to prepare it. At your nearest Asian food store, you will find it.

- With the provided directions, prepare this in your Instant Pot or slow cooker. If required, you may use heavy whipping cream for coconut milk.

3. JALAPENO POPPER SOUP

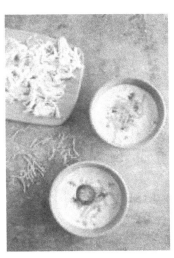

Serving: 3

Preparation time: 25 minutes

Nutritional values: 446kcal Calories | 35g Fat | 4g Carbs | 28g Proteins

Ingredients

- 4 bacon strips
- 2 spoonful's of butter
- Medium-sized 1/2 onion, chopped
- 1/4 cup of pickled, diced jalapenos
- 2 cups broth of chicken
- 2 cups of shredded chicken, cooked
- Cream cheese 4 ounces
- Heavy cream 1/3 cup
- 1 cup of Fresh Cheddar Shredded
- 1/4 tsp. powdered garlic
- Pepper and salt, to taste
- If needed, 1/2 tsp. xanthan gum for thick soup [Optional]

Directions

1. Fry the bacon in a pan. Crumble when cooked and put aside. Place a large pot over the moderate flame while the bacon cooks. Include the onion and butter and simmer until the onion becomes porous.

2. Transfer the jalapenos and half the crumbled bacon to the pot.

3. Pour in the broth of the chicken and the shredded chicken. Take to a boil, then cook for 20 minutes, and reduce.

4. Put the cream cheese in a medium bowl and microwave for around 20 seconds; once soft until smooth, mix. Stir the cream cheese and the heavy cream into the soup. It may take a few minutes for the cream cheese to be completely integrated. Turn the heat off.

5. Include the shredded cheese, and whisk until it is completely melted. Add xanthan gum at this stage if the thick soup is preferred.

6. Serve with the leftover bacon on top.

4. PEPPERS & SAUSAGES

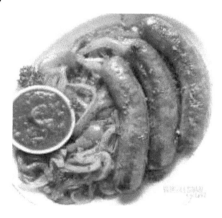

Serving: 6
Preparation time: 2 hrs.5 minutes
Nutritional values: 313kcal Calories | 22g Fat | 11g Carbs | 16g Proteins
Ingredients

- 1 tablespoon olive oil
- Six medium links of Pork sausage
- 3 of the large Bell peppers (cut into strips)
- 1 onion of large size (cut into half, the same size as the pepper shreds)
- Garlic 6 Cloves (minced)
- 1 tbsp. seasoning Italian
- Sea salt about 1/2 tsp.

- Black pepper 1/4 teaspoon
- 1 and a half cups of Marinara sauce

Directions

1. To activate a kitchen timer whilst you cook, toggle on the times in the directions below.

2. Heat the oil over moderate heat in a large pan. Include the sausage links until its warm. Cook on either side for around 2 minutes, only until golden brown on the outer side. (Inside, they will not be prepared.)

3. In the meantime, in a slow cooker, add the bell peppers, onions, garlic, Italian spices, salt, & pepper. Toss it to coat it. Softly spill the marinara sauce over the veggies.

4. Once the sausage links are golden brown, put them on top of the veggies in the slow cooker.

5. Cook on low flame or 2-3 hours on high flame for 4-5 hours, unless the sausages are cooked completely.

5. SHRIMPS WITH CAULIFLOWER GRITS AND ARUGULA

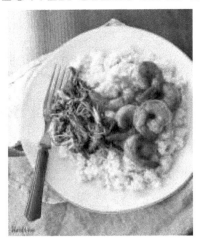

Serving: 4

Preparation time: 25-30 minutes

Nutritional values: 123kcal Calories | 5g Fat | 3g Carbs | 16g proteins

Ingredients

For Spicy Shrimp

- 1 pound of cleaned and roasted shrimp
- 1 tablespoon of paprika
- 2 teaspoons of powdered garlic
- 1/2 tsp. of pepper cayenne
- 1 tablespoon of olive oil extra virgin
- Salt and black pepper freshly processed
- GRITS of CAULIFLOWER
- Unsalted butter about 1 tablespoon
- Riced cauliflower about four cups
- 1cup of milk
- 1/2 cup of goat's crushed cheese
- Salt & black pepper freshly processed

For Garlic Arugula

- 1 tablespoon of olive oil extra virgin
- 3 cloves of garlic, finely minced
- 4 cups of baby arugula
- Salt & black pepper freshly processed

Directions

1. **Prepare the Spicy Shrimp:** Put the shrimp in a big plastic zip-top pack. Mix the paprika in a tiny bowl with the garlic powder as well as the cayenne to blend. Place the mixture with the shrimp into the packet and shake well before the spices have covered them. Refrigerate the grits while preparing them.

2. **Prepare the Cauliflower "Grits":** Melt the butter over a moderate flame in a wide bowl. Integrate the cauliflower rice and simmer for 2 to 3 minutes once it sheds some of its steam.

3. Whisk in half the milk and raise it to a boil. Continue to boil, stirring regularly, for 6 to 8 minutes, before some milk is consumed by the cauliflower.

4. Add the leftover milk and boil for another 10 minutes before the mixture is smooth and fluffy. Mix in the cheese from the goat and add salt and pepper. Just hold warm.

5. **Prepare Garlic Arugula:** Warm olive oil over moderate heat in a large pan. Add the garlic and simmer for 1 minute unless tangy. Include the arugula and simmer for 3 to 4 minutes, unless softened. Use salt and pepper to season, take from the pan, and put aside.

6. Heat the olive oil over low heat in the same pan. Include shrimp and simmer for 4 to 5 minutes until completely cooked. Use salt and pepper to season.

7. Divide the grits into four dishes to serve, then top each one with a fourth of the arugula & a quarter of the shrimp. Immediately serve.

6. CHICKEN CHILI WHITE

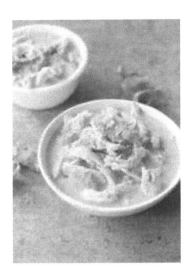

Serving: 4

Preparation time: 35-45 minutes

Nutritional values: 481kcal Calories | 30g Fat | 5g Carbs | 39g Proteins

Ingredients

- 1 lb. breast of chicken
- Chicken broth about 1.5 cups
- 2 cloves of garlic, thinly chopped
- 1 can of sliced green chills
- 1 jalapeno sliced
- 1 green pepper chopped
- 1/4 cup onion finely chopped
- Four tablespoons of butter
- 1/4 cup of heavy whipped cream
- Four-ounce cream cheese
- 2 teaspoons of cumin
- 1 teaspoon of oregano
- Cayenne 1/4 teaspoon (additional)
- To taste: salt & black pepper

Directions

1. Season the chicken with cumin, cayenne, oregano, salt, and black pepper in a wide pan.

2. Braise both sides unless golden, under medium-high heat,

3. Transfer the broth to the pan, cover, and cook for 15-20 minutes or until the chicken is completely cooked.

4. Melt the butter in a moderate pan while the chicken is frying.

5. In the pan, incorporate the chills, chopped jalapeno, green pepper, and onion, and simmer until the vegetables soften.

6. Add the chopped garlic and simmer for an extra 30 seconds, switching off the heat and put aside.

7. When the chicken is fully done, slice it with a fork and transfer it to the broth.

8. In a chicken & broth pan, incorporate the sautéed veggies and cook for 10 minutes.

9. Soften the cream cheese in the microwave in a mixing bowl so you can blend it (~20 sec)

10. Mix the cream cheese and heavy whipped cream

11. Add the mixture of chicken and vegetables into the pot and whisk rapidly.

12. Simmer for an extra 15 minutes.

13. Serve with preferred toppings such as cheese from the pepper jack, slices of avocado, coriander, sour cream.

7. BOWL OF CHICKEN ENCHILADA

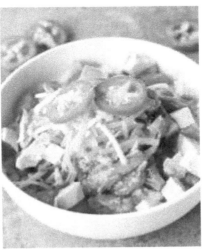

Serving: 4

Preparation time: 40-50 minutes

Nutritional values: 570kcal Calories | 40g Fat | 6g Carbs | 38g Proteins

Ingredients

- 2 spoonful's of coconut oil (for searing chicken)
- 1 pound of chicken thighs that are boneless, skinless
- 3/4 cup sauce of red enchilada
- 1/4 of a cup of water
- 1/4 cup onion, minced
- 1-4 oz. green chills Can - sliced

Toppings

- 1 Avocado, sliced
- 1 cup of cheese, crushed
- 1/4 cup of pickled jalapenos, diced
- 1/2 of a cup of sour cream
- 1 tomato Roma, diced

Directions

1. Heat up the coconut oil on a moderate flame in a pan or a Dutch oven. Braise the chicken thighs unless finely brown when hot.

2. Place in the enchilada sauce as well as the water. After this, add the onion and also the green chilies. Lower the heat to a boil and cover it. Cook the chicken for 17-25 minutes or until the chicken is juicy and heated to an inner temperature of approximately 165 degrees.

3. Remove the chicken cautiously and put it on a chopping board. Then put it back into the pot. Cut or shred chicken (your preference). To retain flavor, let the chicken boil uncovered for an extra 10 minutes and enable the sauce to minimize some more.

4. For serving, cover with avocado, cheese, jalapeno, tomato, sour cream, or any other toppings you want. Feel free to adjust them to your taste. If preferred, serve individually or over cauliflower rice; just refresh your personal nutrition details as required.

8. CHIPOTLE HEALTHY KETO PULLED PORK

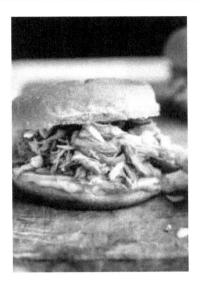

Serving: 10

Preparation time: 8 hrs.15 minutes

Nutritional values: 430kcal Calories | 34g Fat | 3g Carbs | 27g Proteins

Ingredients

- 1 Mid-yellow onion chopped
- 1 cup of water
- 2 tablespoons of fresh garlic diced
- 1 tablespoon of Coconut Sugar
- 1 tablespoon of salt
- 1 teaspoon of chili powder
- 1/2 teaspoon of cumin powder
- 1/2 Tablespoon Adobo sauce
- Smoked paprika 1/4 teaspoons
- 3 1/2-4 lbs. pork shoulder, Extra fat should be removed
- Whole wheat or hamburger buns without gluten OR salad wraps for serving
- Paleo ranch, to be garnished
- Coleslaw blend for optional garnish
- Lime Juice, to be garnished
- Green Tabasco for garnishing

Directions

1. Cut the onion and chop the garlic, and put it in the base of the slow cooker — a spill in a cup of water.

2. In a small bowl, mix all the ingredients for the seasoning and set it aside.

3. Slice off the pork shoulder some large, noticeable parts of fat and spread it all over with the seasoning until it is uniformly covered.

4. Over the top of the garlic, onions & water, add the pork and simmer until soft and juicy, 6-8 hours on maximum or 8-10 hours on reduced.

5. If the pork is cooked, extract much of the liquid from the crockpot and put the solids directly into the crockpot (which comprises the garlic and onions).

6. On a chopping board, move the pork and slice it with two forks.

7. In the slow cooker, shift the sliced pork back and combine with the onions and garlic. Cover unless ready to be served, and keep it warm.

8. On a bun or lettuce, place the pulled pork, served with a ranch coleslaw blend and a pinch of lime juice as well as green tabasco.

9. Enjoy.

9. STIR FRY ZOODLE

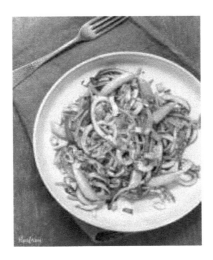

Serving: 4

Preparation time: 15-22 minutes

Nutritional values: 113kcal Calories | 3g Fat | 20g Carbs | 6g Proteins

Ingredients

- Sesame oil 11/2 tsp. (or 1 tbsp. of olive oil)
- 1 bunch of thinly chopped scallions
- 2 cloves of garlic, chopped
- 1 tablespoon of fresh ginger, diced
- Two carrots, chopped into thin strands
- One red pepper bell, cut into small strands,
- Two cups of snap peas
- Four zucchini, sliced into noodles (using a utensil like this)
- 1/4 cup of soy sauce
- 3 tbsp. vinegar for rice
- 1/4 cup of fresh cilantro, diced

Directions

1. Add the oil in a wide sauté pan over medium heat. Integrate the scallions, garlic, and ginger and simmer for 1 to 2 minutes, unless aromatic.

2. Include the bell pepper, carrots, snap peas & zucchini noodles. Sauté for 5 to 6 minutes until the vegetables just start to become soft.

3. Integrate the soy sauce & rice vinegar and proceed to cook unless the vegetables are quite soft and juicy, frequently tossing, for another 3 to 4 minutes.

4. Seasoned with cilantro, serve hot.

10. TEX MEX CHICKEN SALAD

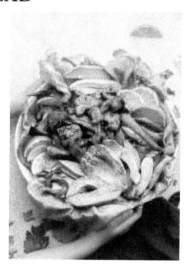

Serving: 4

Preparation time: 25 minutes

Nutritional values: 546kcal Calories | 41g Fat | 12g Carbs | 30g Proteins

Ingredients

- For the seasoning of the fajita:
- 2 tsp. of powdered chili
- 1 tsp. of cumin
- 1 tsp. of powdered garlic
- 1 teaspoon powdered onion
- 1 tsp. of paprika. smoked
- 1/2 tsp. of or to taste salt

For the fajitas

- Two spoonful's of olive oil
- 1/2 tsp. ground mustard OR 1 tbsp. of Dijon mustard as required
- 1 lemon juice
- 2 medium breasts of chicken hammered to even density
- 2 tablespoons divided butter
- 4 finely diced medium bell peppers into slices
- 1 medium red onion finely sliced into slices

- 2-3 leaves of buttered lettuce
- 2-3 leaves of romaine lettuce

To serve
- Slices of lime
- Avocado sliced

Directions

1. Mix all the ingredients for the condiments in a tiny compostable jar. Enclose well and squish. For bell peppers, save 1 1/2 tsp.

2. Integrate two tbsp. of olive oil, lemon juice, and 5 tsp. of fajita condiments in a wide, zip lock bag. In the bag, add the chicken and secure it. Push the marinade into the chicken and enable the vegetables to marinate while preparing them (or freeze in the fridge unless ready to use).

3. Cut the bell peppers as well as onions.

4. Heat 1 tbsp. of butter over moderate heat in a large skillet. Add the onions and cook for approximately 4-5 minutes, or until tender and succulent. Transfer the bell peppers and squirt 1 1/2 tsp. of fajita condiments with the restrained ones. Cook for almost 3-5 minutes if you like the peppers with a lovely crunch. And if you like it softer, end up leaving it on for about two to three minutes long. Set aside and move to a plate.

5. Melt 1 residual tablespoon of butter and brown the chicken in the same pan. Cook for 5-6 minutes, or until properly cooked.

6. In a wide salad bowl or tray, organize the lettuce and top it with chicken as well as bell peppers. Add your chosen sliced avocados, lime slices, and any other seasonings.

11. KETO BROCCOLI CHEDDAR SOUP

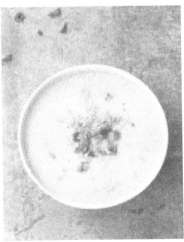

Serving: 4

Preparation time: 20 minutes

Nutritional values: 285kcal Calories | 25g Fat | 3g Carbs | 12g Proteins

Ingredients

- 2 spoonful's of butter
- 1/8 cup of onion, white
- 1/2 tsp. of finely chopped garlic
- 2 cups of broth of chicken
- Pepper and salt, to taste
- 1 cup of broccoli, cut into bite-sized pieces
- 1 spoon of cream cheese
- Heavy whipping cream 1/4 cup
- 1 cup of cheddar cheese, crushed
- Bacon 2 loaves, cooked and Imploded (Optional)
- 1/2 tsp. of gum xanthan (Optional)

Directions

1. Simmer the onion and garlic with butter in a wide pot over medium heat until the onions are seamless and textured.
2. Add broth as well as broccoli to the pot. Until soft, cook broccoli. Add the salt, pepper, and seasoning you want.
3. Put the cream cheese in a medium bowl and heat for ~30 seconds in the microwave until smooth and easy to mix.
4. Mix in the soup with heavy whipping cream and cream cheese; bring to the boil.
5. Turn off the heat and mix the cheddar cheese swiftly.
6. If required, stir in the xanthan gum. Allow for stiffening.
7. Serve hot with implodes of bacon (if desired)

12. SPICY THAI BUTTERNUT SQUASH SOUP

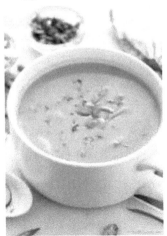

Serving: 4

Preparation time: 30 minutes

Nutritional values: 450kcal Calories | 35g Fat | 35g Carbs | 8g proteins

Ingredients

- 1 1/2 tbsp. coconut oil, refined
- 1 large onion, yellow, sliced
- 1/4 cup of a paste of red curry
- One 2-inch slice of grated or finely chopped garlic
- Four teaspoons of cloves of garlic, diced
- 4 cups vegetable stock with low sodium or water
- 1 peeled and finely diced medium butternut squash (about 4 1/2 cups)
- One 13.5-ounce coconut milk full-fat can
- 1/4 cup cashew butter or almond butter in natural form
- Lower tamari 1 tbsp.
- 1 tablespoon maple syrup or nectar of Agave
- Kosher salt about 1 tsp., plus more to flavor
- Three teaspoons of freshly pressed lemon juice
- 1/2 cup of fresh, chopped cilantro, plus more for garnishing
- Serve with coconut yogurt, roasted peanuts, scallions & sesame seeds

Directions

1. Choose the Instant Pot Sauté mode, then add the coconut oil after several minutes. When the oil is warm, add a bit of salt to the onion, and then cook

for 6 to 7 minutes before it starts to brown. Transfer the curry paste, ginger, and garlic; simmer for about 1 minute, constantly stirring, until quite tangy.

2. Spill the stock in and use a wooden spoon on the bottom of the pot to pick off some browned pieces. Stir in butternut squash, coconut milk, tamari, salt, cashew butter, and maple syrup. To blend properly, mix.

3. Shield the cover and seal the pressure release. Choose the high-pressure setting for the soup and specify the cooking time to 12 minutes.

4. Enable an organic pressure release for 5 minutes when the timer goes off, and then undergo a speedy pressure release.

5. Open the pot, add the lime juice and mix. Mix, so you have a nice and creamy broth using an electric mixer. Conversely, using a dish towel to shield the mixer cap to keep steam from spreading, you should pass the broth in batches to a mixer.

6. Stir in the minced cilantro until the broth is pureed — seasoning with coconut yogurt, peanuts, sesame seeds, and scallions as needed.

13. KETO PHO RECIPE

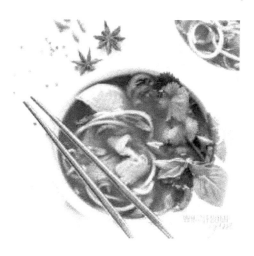

Serving: 4

Preparation time: 35 minutes

Nutritional values: 220kcal Calories | 5g Fat | 8g Carbs | 33g Proteins

Ingredients

- 4 Entire Star Anise
- 2 entire pods of Cardamom
- 2 entire sticks of Cinnamon
- 2 Whole Cloves
- 1 tbsp. seeds of Coriander

- 1 tsp. of ginger
- 8 cups of bone broth of beef
- 1 tablespoon of Fish sauce
- 1 tbsp. Allulose Mix of Besti Monk Fruit (optional, to taste)
- Salt (optional, to taste)

Soup Pho:

- Flank steak 12 oz. (trimmed, or sirloin)
- 2 large Zucchinis (spiraled into zoodles)

Pho toppings optional:

- Thai basil
- Cilantro
- Wedges of lime
- Slices of red chili pepper (or jalapeno peppers)
- Scallions
- Sriracha

Directions

1. For 30 minutes, put the steak in the refrigerator to make it easy to slice finely.

2. In the meantime, over moderate heat, warm a Dutch oven, minus oil. Bring the star anise, pods of cardamom, sticks of cinnamon, garlic, seeds of coriander, and fresh ginger. Toast, until aromatic, for 2-3 minutes.

3. Combine the fish sauce as well as bone broth. Mix together—Cook the pho broth and stew for 30 minutes.

4. In the meantime, to make zoodles out from the zucchini, use a spiralizer. Split the noodles from the zucchini into 4 bowls.

5. Pull it out and slice rather thinly against the grain until the steak in the refrigerator is stable. Put the steak inside each bowl on top of the zoodles.

6. Mix in the sweetener to disintegrate (if used) and modify the salt to taste whenever the broth is finished simmering. In a different pot or bowl, extract the soup. Discard all the spices that are trapped in the strainer.

7. Although the broth is already simmering, spill it over the preparing bowls instantly, making sure that the steak is immersed, so it cooks completely. (Conversely, the steak should first be stirred into the boiling broth.)

8. Thai basil, coriander, lemon slices, jalapeno or chili pepper strips, scallions, and Sriracha, and garnish with condiments of you're choosing.

14. PORK CARNITAS

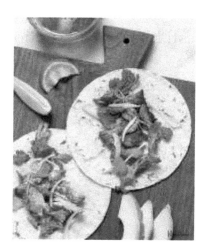

Serving: 8

Preparation time: 7 hrs.15 min

Nutritional values: 442kcal Calories | 31g Fat | 9g Carbs30g Proteins

Ingredients

- 1 white, halved, and finely chopped onion
- Five cloves of garlic, chopped
- 1 jalapeño, chopped,
- 3 lbs. of cubed shoulder pork
- Salt and black pepper finely ground
- 1 tablespoon of cumin
- 2 tbsp. of fresh oregano minced
- Two Oranges
- 1 lemon
- 1/3 cup of broth of chicken

Directions

1. At the base of a slow cooker, put the onion, jalapeño garlic, pork together. Add the salt, pepper, oregano & cumin.

2. The oranges and lime are zested over the pork, then halved, and the juice is squeezed over the pork. Also, spill the broth over the pork.

3. Put the cover on and adjust the heat to medium on the slow cooker. Process for 7 hours or unless the meat is soft and quick to squash with a fork.

4. Shred the pork with two forks. The pork may be eaten instantly or frozen in an airtight jar for up to 5 days in the fridge or for up to one month in the freezer.

15. CHICKEN MEATBALLS AND CAULIFLOWER RICE WITH COCONUT HERB SAUCE

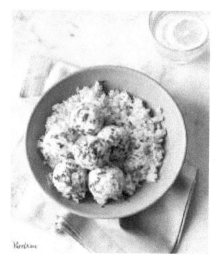

Serving: 4

Preparation time: 45 minutes

Nutritional values: 205kcal calories | 13g Fat | 3g Carbs | 20g Proteins

Ingredients

For meatballs

- Non-stick spray
- 1 tablespoon of extra virgin olive oil
- 1/2 of the red onion
- 2 cloves of garlic, chopped
- 1 lb. of ground chicken
- 1/4 cup of finely minced parsley
- 1 tablespoon of Dijon mustard
- 3/4 tsp. of kosher salt
- 1/2 tsp. of freshly ground black pepper

For sauce

- One 14-ounce of coconut milk can
- 11/4 cups of fresh, chopped parsley, distributed
- Four scallions, minced roughly
- 1 clove of garlic, peeled and crushed
- Juice and zest of one lime

- Kosher salt and black pepper, recently ground
- Red pepper flakes to serve.
- 1 Cauliflower Rice recipe

Directions

1. **Prepare the meatballs:** Set the oven to 375°F. Cover a baking sheet with aluminum foil and coat it with a non-stick spray.
2. Heat the oil in a wide skillet over medium heat. Integrate the onion and simmer until soft, about five minutes. Integrate the garlic and simmer until tangy for around 1 minute.
3. Shift the onion and garlic to a mixing saucepan and let it cool completely. Mix in chicken, parsley, and mustard, sprinkle with salt. Turn the paste into 2 tablespoon balls and shift to the parchment paper.
4. Cook the meatballs for 17 to 20 minutes until firm and fully cooked.
5. **Prepare the sauce:** In a food processor pan, blend coconut milk, scallions, parsley, garlic, lime juice & lemon zest and stir unless buttery; season with salt and pepper.
6. Cover with the red pepper flakes as well as the leftover parsley. With the sauce, end up serving over the cauliflower rice.

16. KETO RAINBOW VEGGIES AND SHEET PAN CHICKEN

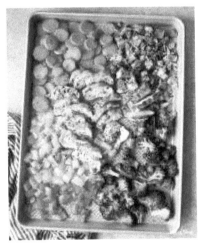

Serving: 4

Preparation time: 40 minutes

Nutritional values: 380kcal Calories | 14g Fat | 35g Carbs | 31g Proteins

Ingredients

- Spray for Nonstick

- 1 lb. of boneless chicken breasts without skin
- Sesame Oil 1 tbsp.
- 2 spoonful's of soy sauce
- Honey about 2 tablespoons
- 2 bell peppers, red, chopped
- 2 bell peppers yellow, chopped
- Three carrots, diced
- 1/2 broccoli head, sliced into cloves
- 2 red, chopped onions
- Extra virgin olive oil about 2 tablespoons
- Kosher salt and black pepper, recently ground
- 1/4 cup of fresh parsley, minced, for serving

Directions

1. Heat up the oven to 400 degrees F. Slather a baking sheet lightly with non - stick spray.

2. Put the chicken on the baking tray. Stir the sesame oil and soy sauce together in a medium bowl. Dust the blend over the chicken equally.

3. On the baking dish, place the red and yellow bell peppers, broccoli, carrot & red onion. Sprinkle over the vegetables with olive oil and softly toss to coat; season with salt and pepper.

4. Roast it for 23 to 25 minutes until the veggies are soft and the chicken is thoroughly cooked. Take it out of the oven and seasoned it with parsley.

17. CAULIFLOWER POTATO SALAD

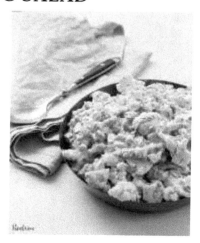

Serving: 6

Preparation time: 30-40 minutes

Nutritional values: 90kcal Calories | 4g Fat | 9g Carbs | 5g Proteins

Ingredients

- 1 head cauliflower, sliced into chunks that are bite-sized
- 3/4 cup of Greek yogurt
- 1/4 cup of sour cream
- 1 tbsp. Mustard from Dijon
- 2 tbsp. apple cider vinegar
- 1 tablespoon of fresh parsley minced
- 1 tbsp. fresh dill minced
- Celery 4 stalks, finely chopped
- 1 bunch of green, finely chopped onions
- 1/3 cup of cornichons diced
- Kosher salt and black pepper, freshly processed

Directions

1. Put the cauliflower, then coat it with water in a large container. Take the cauliflower to a simmer over moderate flame and boil until it is just fork soft, 8 to 10 minutes (do not overcook it, because, in the salad, it may not keep up).

2. Gently soak and cool the cauliflower to normal temperature. Meanwhile, mix the Greek yogurt, sour cream, mustard, vinegar, parsley, and dill together in a wide cup.

3. To incorporate, add the cauliflower, celery, green onions, and cornichons to the bowl and mix well. Sprinkle with salt & pepper.

4. When eating, chill the salad for a minimum of 1 hour. It is possible to prepare the salad 1 day in advance and keep it in the fridge until ready to eat.

18. PROSCIUTTO WRAPPED CAULIFLOWER BITES

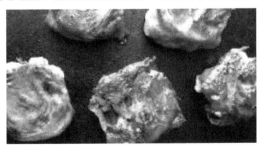

Serving: 8-10

Preparation time: 15 minutes

Nutritional values: 215kcal Calories | 15g Fat | 5g Carbs | 15g Proteins

Ingredients

- 1 tiny cauliflower
- 1/2 cup of paste of tomatoes
- 2 spoonful's of white wine
- 1/2 tsp. of black pepper
- 1/2 cup of Parmesan cheese grated
- 20 Prosciutto slices
- 6 tbsp. of extra-virgin olive oil

Directions

1. Start preparing the cauliflower: Cut the base, and any green leaves, away from the cauliflower. Halve the cauliflower, and slice the halves into 1-inch-thick pieces. Based on the size of the slice, divide the slices into 2 or 3 bite-size bits.

2. Bring a big saucepan of salted water to a boil. In the water, parboil the cauliflower until almost soft, for 3 to 5 minutes. With paper towels, rinse the cauliflower well enough and pat off.

3. Add the tomato paste with the white wine & black pepper in a small dish to blend. On the edges of each slice of cauliflower, distribute 1 tsp., then dust with 1 tsp. of Parmesan. A prosciutto slice is carefully wrapped over each piece of cauliflower, pushing softly at the edge to seal it (it should twig well to the tomato-paste blend).

4. Continuing to work in chunks, heat two tablespoons of olive oil over moderate heat in a large pan. Add the cauliflower while the oil is hot and simmer unless the prosciutto is crispy and golden, 3 to 4 minutes on either

side. Repeat till all the pieces are ready, with extra oil and cauliflower. Let it cool slowly, then serve right away.

19. CAULIFLOWER TORTILLAS

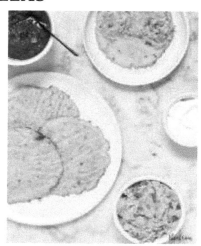

Serving: 6

Preparation time: 45 minutes

Nutritional values: 45kcal Calories | 2g Fat | 5g Carbs | 4g Proteins

Ingredients

- 1 head cauliflower
- 2 eggs, pounded lightly
- 1/2 tsp. cumin
- 1/4 tsp. of cayenne pepper
- Salt and black pepper, freshly processed, to taste

Directions

1. Heat up the oven to 375°F. Use parchment paper to cover a baking sheet.

2. Split the cauliflower into thin strips. Cut the delicate portion of the stems roughly (discard the tough and leafy parts).

3. Move the cauliflower to the mixing bowl, filling it just halfway, working in bundles. Compress the cauliflower until it looks like rice, around 45 seconds to 1 minute. Repeat for the cauliflower that remains.

4. Move the cauliflower to a dish that is microwave-safe. Microwave around 1 minute, mix well, and microwave for an extra 1 minute.

5. Move the cauliflower to a tidy kitchen towel in the center. In a twist, cover the cauliflower up. Keep the towel over the basin and curl the ends to suck the humidity out of the cauliflower.

6. Take the cauliflower back to the bowl. Add the eggs, cumin, cayenne, salt, and black pepper, and mix well.

7. Ridge the lined baking sheet with 1/4 cup of cauliflower scoops. Distribute the cauliflower into 1/8-inch-thick circles using a tiny spoon.

8. For around 8 to 9 minutes, cook the tortillas until the bottoms are crispy. Then use a spatula to turn the tortillas over cautiously and cook for another 8 to 9 minutes unless crispy on the other side.

9. The tortillas can be eaten hot, instantly, or frozen for up to five days in an airtight jar in the fridge (with parchment pieces among them).

20. KETO SALMON SUSHI BOWL

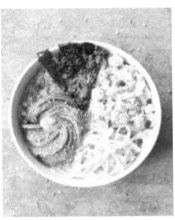

Serving: 3-4

Preparation time: 15 minutes

Nutritional values: 45kcal Calories | 6g Fat | 8g Carbs | 9g Proteins

Ingredients

- Cauliflower Rice 3/4 Cup
- Smoked salmon about 1/2 packet
- 1/2 cup of cucumber spiraled
- Avocado 1/2
- 2 sheets of seaweed-dried
- 1 teaspoon of low sodium soy sauce
- Pepper & salt, to taste
- Wasabi 1/2 teaspoon, optional

Sauce

- 3 tbsp. mayonnaise
- Sriracha 1-2 teaspoon (adjust to preference)

Direction

1. Steam the cauliflower rice and incorporate salt and black pepper (I used premade bag)
2. Put the rice layer with soy sauce as well as seasoning in the bottom of the small dish.
3. Fill the bowl with salmon, cucumber, seaweed, and avocado
4. Integrate mayo and Sriracha for sauce, adapting to the preferred heat.
5. Spread the sauce over a dish.
6. If desired, add sesame seeds as well as pepper for garnishing.

2.3 Keto Snacks

1. BAKED GARLIC PARMESAN ZUCCHINI CHIPS

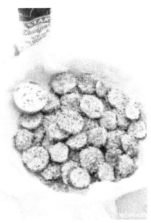

Serving: 6

Preparation time: 20-30 minutes

Nutritional values: 155kcal Calories | 10g Fat | 10g Carbs | 5g Proteins

Ingredients

- Chopped 3 to 4 zucchini into pieces of 1/4-inch and 1/2-inch
- 3 tbsp. of Omega-3 DHA Extra Virgin Olive Oil STAR
- Salt to taste and freshly ground pepper
- 1 cup bread crumbs of panko
- 1/2- cup of Parmesan grated cheese
- 1 tsp. of oregano that is dried
- 1 tsp. of powdered garlic
- Cooking spray
- Non-Fat simple yogurt, for serving,

Directions

1. Preheat the cooking oven to 450.
2. Line 3 foil-based baking sheets; brush lightly with cooking spray, then set it aside.
3. Incorporate the zucchini pieces, olive oil, salt, and pepper in a wide mixing bowl; whisk until well mixed.
4. Incorporate the crumbs, cheese, oregano, plus garlic powder in a different dish.

5. Dip the zucchini pieces in the cheese mixture and cover on both ends, press to remain with the coating.

6. On the prepared baking sheets, put the slices of zucchini in a thin layer.

7. Spray every slice lightly with cooking spray. This would help to achieve a texture that is crispier.

8. Flip the pan and finish frying for 8 - 10 mints, or until the chips are nicely browned — bake for ten min.

9. Remove it from the oven.

10. With Non-Fat Simple Yogurt, serve it.

2. KETO PIZZA ROLL-UPS

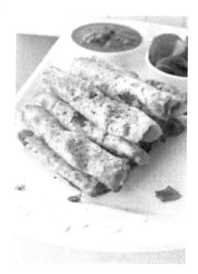

Serving: 8-10

Preparation time: 15 minutes

Nutritional values: 138kcal Calories | 12g Fat | 8g Carbs | 6g Proteins

Ingredients

- 12 mozzarella cheese slices
- Chunks of pepperoni, or you may use small pepperoni as well.
- Seasoning - Italian
- Marina Sauce - Keto

Directions

1. Heat the oven to 400°F.

2. Using a baking mat and parchment paper, cover a cookie sheet.

3. Position the slices of cheese on the baking mat, then place them in the oven for 6 mints, or unless the slices of cheese tend to brown across the corners.

4. Take it out from the oven and leave to cool the cheese moderately. If you like, make the slices to chill and scatter with Italian seasoning, as well as include pepperoni.

5. With your chosen dipping sauce, wrap & serve! Enjoy

3. STUFFED MUSHROOMS WITH SAUSAGE

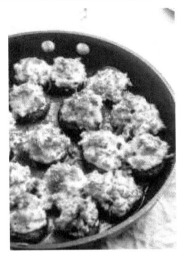

Serving: 8

Preparation time: 30-40 minutes

Nutritional values: 280kcal Calories | 20g Fat | 6g Carbs | 15g Proteins

Ingredients

- 1 pound of mild Italian sausage
- Cremini mushrooms about 1 pound
- 4 ounces of cream cheese
- 1/3 cup mozzarella - shredded
- Salt, as necessary
- ½ Teaspoon flakes of red pepper
- 1/4 cup of Parmesan grated cheese

Directions

1. To 350F, set the oven. Wash and cut the stems from the mushrooms.

2. Cook the sausage in a wide skillet over moderate heat. Transfer it to a wide mixing bowl until it has been cooked.

3. Add the mozzarella cheese, cream cheese, and mix to combine. Season to taste, then add salt & red pepper if required.

4. Spoon onto the mushroom caps with the sausage combination. Use Parmesan cheese for scattering. Put in a pan or casserole platter that is oven-safe.

5. Bake for 25 mints, unless the cheese is golden brown and the mushrooms are tender.

4. EASY KETO PIZZA BITES

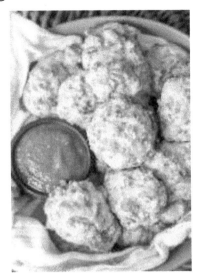

Serving: 30

Preparation time: 30-35 minutes

Nutritional values: 82kcal Calories | 7g Fat | 1g Carbs | 4g Proteins

Ingredients

- 1 lb., cooked as well as drained Italian sausage
- Cream cheese, 4 ounces, softened.
- 1/3 of a cup of cocoa flour
- 1/2 tsp. powder for baking
- 1 tsp. of garlic diced
- 1 tsp. of seasoning - Italian
- 3 large, beaten eggs
- 1 1/4 cup mozzarella crushed

Directions

1. Preheat the oven to 350°F.
2. Mix the prepared sausage & cream cheese unless fully fused together.
3. To give the flour time to ponder the moisture, rest of the ingredients until well mixed and cool for 10 minutes.
4. If you forget to chill the dough, they will deflate while they cook and will not be pleasant round balls.
5. Use a tiny cookie scoop to transfer onto a greased baking sheet (I prefer using the silicone baking mats).

6. Bake until lightly browned for 18-20 minutes.

7. This made 30, so it depends on the scale of the scoop you're using and how closely you're packing it.

5. CUCUMBER SLICES WITH HERB AND GARLIC CHEESE

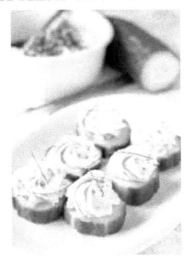

Serving: 16

Preparation time: 5 minutes

Nutritional values: 42kcal Calories | 3g Fat | 1g Carbs | 1g Proteins

Ingredients

- 1 Diced English cucumber into 16 slices
- The Chives
- 6.5 ounces of Boursin or Alouette Herb & Garlic Cheese

Directions

1. To include some novelty, cut short slices of the cucumber skin with the help of a vegetable peeler.
2. Cut the cucumber to a thickness of around 1 mm.
3. Put the cheese in a pastry bag equipped with the edge of a large star.
4. The cucumber tips could clear every moister with a paper towel pat.
5. Puff each cucumber with the cheese and cover with a piece of chives.

6. KETO POPCORN - PUFFED CHEESE

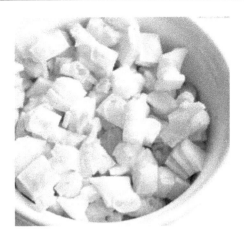

Serving: 5

Preparation: 10 minutes

Nutritional values: 80kcal Calories | 7g Fat | 0.3g Carbs | 5g Proteins

Ingredients

- cheddar 100g/3.5 ounces

Directions

1. Slice the cheese into 0.5 inches / 1 cm pieces if you use diced cheddar. If you are using a block of cheddar, crush it to the same size using your fingertips.

2. Use a cloth/kitchen towel to wrap the cheese to keep it from being gritty and let it stay for up to 3 days in a hot, dry spot. You would like the cheese to be solid and dried absolutely.

3. Preheat oven to 390 Fahrenheit / 200 Celsius. On a baking tray covered with parchment paper, spread the cheese and bake for 4-five minutes before the cheese bursts. Put a new baking tray securely over the tray to keep it from popping out over the oven.

7. BACON WRAPPED BRUSSELS SPROUTS

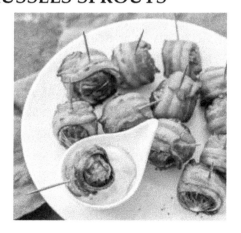

Serving: 4

Preparation time: 40 minutes

Nutritional values: 170kcal Calories | 15g Fat | 3g Carbs | 2g Proteins

Ingredients

12 bacon slices

12 Brussels sprouts, cut stems

Balsamic Dip:

Mayonnaise 5 tbsp.

Balsamic vinegar about 1 tbsp.

Directions

1. Preparation: Set aside baking sheets and 12 toothpicks, covered with parchment paper or a baking mat that would be non-stick—preheat the baking oven to 400 F.

2. Wrap Sprouts: Put 1 slice of bacon on each sprout of Brussels, seal it with a toothpick, and put on the baking sheet in a thin layer.

3. Bake: Bake discovered at 400 F until the bacon is translucent and the Brussels are quite juicy around 40 minutes.

4. Serve: In a medium bowl, blend the mayonnaise & balsamic vinegar altogether unless creamy. Serve Brussels sprouts covered with bacon on a plate, along with the dip.

8. KETO ASPARAGUS FRIES

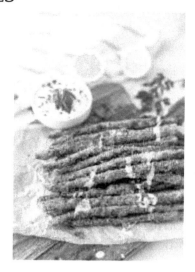

Serving: 6

Preparation time: 1hour

Nutritional values: 202kcal Calories | 14g Fat | 7g Carbs | 14g Proteins

Ingredients

- 1 pound of asparagus chopped (thick if possible)
- Salt and pepper to taste
- 1 cup of Parmesan cheese
- 3/4 cup of almond flour
- 1/4 tsp. of cayenne pepper
- 1/4 tsp. of baking powder
- 4 pounded eggs
- avocado oil spray

Directions

1. Use a fork to cut the asparagus spikes with gaps—season well with a minimum of 1/2 teaspoon of salt. Put on paper towels and let it rest for 30 minutes.

2. In the meantime, mix 1 cup of Parmesan, cayenne pepper, almond flour & baking powder in a dish. Sprinkle with salt to taste.

3. Pound the egg in a different dish.

4. Soak the asparagus segments in the eggs, then cover with the blend of the cheese.

5. Your air fryer should be preheated to 400 degrees.

6. Organize the asparagus in one layer and, if required, cook in chunks. Spray the oil well—Cook for five minutes. Turn, and then respray.

7. Fry unless the asparagus is soft for the next 4 or 5 minutes.

9. EGG, BACON, AND CHEESE SLIDERS

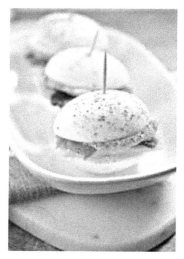

Serving: 6

Preparation time: 10 minutes

Nutritional values: 237kcal Calories | 18g Fat | 3g Carbs | 15g Proteins

Ingredients

- 6 peeled, boiled eggs
- 6 Thin cheddar cheese strips
- 3 Slices of bacon that has been cooked
- 1/2 of Avocado
- 1/2 teaspoon Juice of a lime
- 1/2 Teaspoon cumin

Directions

1. In a mixing bowl, place 1/2 of an avocado.
2. Stir in the cumin as well as lime juice. Mix until completely smooth. To taste, incorporate the salt.
3. Cut each hardboiled egg lengthwise in half.
4. Put on the lower half of the egg one piece of thinly cut cheddar cheese.
5. Place 1/2 a slice of cooked bacon on edge.
6. On the edge of the bacon, put a spoonful of the avocado mixture on top.
7. To make a little sandwich, place the remaining half of the egg face right over the top. Protect the bite of the egg with a toothpick placed down the center.
8. For your remaining eggs, replicate steps 4-7.

9. Add salt and pepper to each bite of the egg to taste & serve.

10. TURKEY BACON WRAP RANCH PINWHEELS

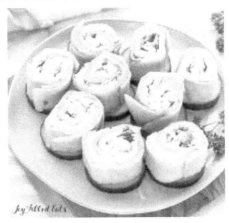

Serving: 6

Preparation time: 15 minutes

Nutritional values: 133kcal Calories | 12g Fat | 2g Carbs | 5g proteins

Ingredients

- 6 ounces of cheese cream
- 12 strips of smoked turkey deli (about 3 oz.)
- 1/4 teaspoon powdered garlic
- 1/4 teaspoon of chopped dried onion
- Dried dill weed 1/4 teaspoon
- 1 tablespoon of crumbling bacon
- 2 tablespoons cheddar shredded cheese

Directions

1. Among 2 pieces of plastic wrap, place the cream cheese. Stretch it out until it's approximately 1/4 inch thick. Scrape the plastic wrap off the top piece. On top of the cream cheese, place the slices of turkey on the edge.

2. Cover and switch the whole item over with a fresh layer of plastic wrap. Chop off the plastic bit that is on the upper right now. Slather it on top of the cream cheese with the seasoning. Spray it with cheese and bacon.

3. Roll the pinwheels up such that the exterior is the turkey. Refrigerate for 2 minimum hours. On the edge of low-carb crackers or diced cucumber, cut into 12 bits and serve.

2.4 Keto Desserts

1. KETO BROWN BUTTER PRALINES

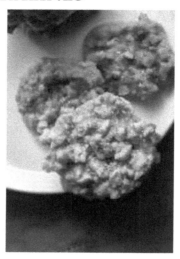

Serving: 10

Preparation time: 16 minutes

Nutritional values: 338kcal Calories | 36g Fat | 3g Carbs | 2g Proteins

Ingredients

- 2 Salted butter sticks
- Heavy cream 2/3 cup
- 2/3 Cup of Sweetener Granular 1/2 tsp. of xanthan gum
- 2 Cups Pecans diced
- Maldon Sea salt

Directions

1. Use parchment paper or a silicone baking mat to make a cookie sheet.

2. Cook the butter in a skillet over medium flame, stirring regularly. It's going to take less than five min. Whisk in the heavy cream, sweetener, and xanthan gum. Extract it from the heat.

3. Mix in the nuts and put in the fridge, stirring regularly, for 1 hour to tighten up. The mixture's going to get really dense. Scrape onto the prepared baking sheet into 10 cookie styles and spray, if necessary, with the Maldon salt. Let the baking sheet freeze until frozen.

4. Store and keep stored in the fridge until served in an airtight dish.

2. KETO CHOCOLATE MOUSSE

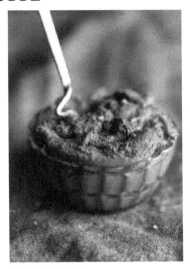

Serving: 4

Preparation time: 10 minutes

Nutritional values: 220kcal Calories | 25g Fat | 5g Carbs | 2g Proteins

Ingredients

- 1 Cup of Whipped Heavy Cream
- 1/4 cup Cocoa powder unsweetened, sifted
- 1/4 Cup Sweetener Powdered
- 1 tsp. extract of vanilla
- Kosher salt about 1/4 teaspoon

Directions

1. Use the cream to whip into stiff peaks. Include the cocoa powder, vanilla, sweetener, and salt, then mix until all the products are mixed.

3. KETO CHEESECAKE FLUFF

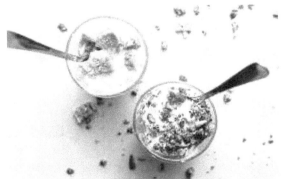

Serving: 6

Preparation time: 10 minutes

Nutritional values: 260kcal Calories | 27g Fat | 4g Carbs | 4g Proteins

Ingredients

- 1 Cup of Whipping Heavy Cream
- 1 Eight oz. Cream Cheese Brick, Softened
- 1 Lemon Zest
- 1/2 Cup of Sweetener Granular

Directions

1. In a stand mixer, combine the heavy cream as well as stir until stiff peaks are made. A hand blender or a whisk can also be used by hand using a whisk.
2. In a different bowl, scrape the whipped cream and put it aside.
3. In the stand blender bowl, add the textured cream cheese, zest, and sweetener, then beat until sturdy.
4. With the cream cheese, add the whipped cream into the stand blender dish. Mix carefully until it is halfway mixed with a spatula. To finish whipping until sturdy, use the stand mixer.
5. Serve with a favorite topping of you.

4. LOW CARB BLUEBERRY CRISP

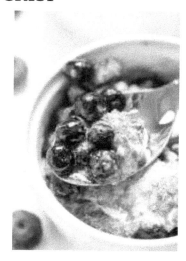

Serving: 2

Preparation time: 20-25 minutes

Nutritional values: 390kcal Calories | 35g Fat | 17g Carbs | 6g Proteins

Ingredients

- 1 Cup of Fresh or Frozen Blueberries
- 1/4 Cup Halves of Pecan

- Almond Meal/Flour 1/8 cup
- Butter around 2 tbsp.
- Granular Sweetener 2 tablespoons - distributed
- 1 tablespoon of flax
- Cinnamon 1/2 Teaspoon
- ½ teaspoon Extract from vanilla
- Kosher salt about 1/4 teaspoon
- Heavy cream 2 tablespoons

Directions

1. Heat the oven to 400F.
2. Put 1/2 cup of blueberries and 1/2 tablespoons of swerve sweetener in 2, 1 cup ramekins. Blend and combine.
3. Incorporate the pecans, almond flour, butter, 1 tbsp. sweetener, cinnamon, ground flax, vanilla, and kosher salt into the food processor. Pulse while you mix the ingredients.
4. Place on top of the blueberries with the blend. Put the ramekins on a baking sheet and cook for 15-20 minutes in the middle of the oven or until the topping turn's toasty brown. Serve with 1 tablespoon of heavy cream slathered on top of each one.

5. 1 MINT LOW CARB BROWNIE

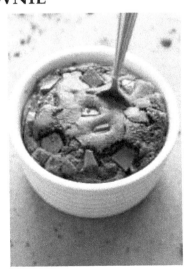

Serving: 1

Preparation time: 3 minutes

Nutritional values: 196kcal Calories | 17g Fat | 2g Carbs | 8g Proteins

Ingredients

- 2 tablespoons almond flour
- 1 tablespoon of preferred granulated sweetener
- 1 tablespoon powdered cocoa
- Baking Powder 1/8 teaspoon
- Almond butter 1 tablespoon. * See notes
- 3 tablespoons of milk, unsweetened almond milk,
- 1 tablespoon of chocolate chips of preference - optional

Directions

1. A tiny microwave-protected cereal bowl or ramkin is lightly greased with cooking spray and placed aside.

2. Integrate all of your dried ingredients in a medium mixing bowl and blend well.

3. Integrate the creamy almond butter and milk in a separate bowl and mix them together. Place the wet and dry ingredients together and blend properly. Roll them through if chocolate chips are used.

4. Microwave at intervals of 30 seconds until the optimal texture has been reached. Take from the microwave then, before eating, let settle for one min.

6. KETO PEANUT BUTTER BALLS

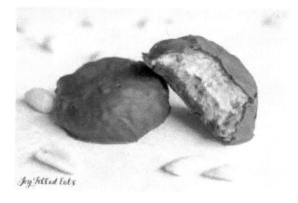

Joy Filled Eats

Serving: 18

Preparation time: 20 minutes

Nutritional values: 195kcal Calories | 17g Fat | 7g Carbs | 7g Proteins

Ingredients

- 1 cup of finely diced salted peanuts (not peanut flour)
- 1 cup of peanut butter

- 1 cup of sweetener powdered, like swerve
- 8-ounce chocolate chips free from sugar

Directions

1. Combine the diced peanuts, peanut butter, and the sweetener, respectively. Distribute the 18-piece crust and mold it into balls. Put them on a baking sheet covered with wax paper. Put it in the fridge until they're cold.

2. In the oven or on top of a dual boiler, heat the chocolate chips. Mix chocolate chips in the microwave, swirling every 30 seconds till they are 75percent melted. Then stir before the remainder of it melts.

3. Soak the chocolate for each peanut butter ball and put it back on the wax paper. Until the chocolate settles, put it in the fridge.

7. WHITE CHOCOLATE PEANUT BUTTER BLONDIES

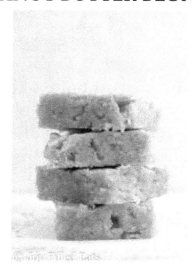

Serving: 16

Preparation time: 35 minutes

Nutritional values: 105kcal Calories | 9g Fat | 2g Carbs | 3g Proteins

Ingredients

- 1/2 cup of peanut butter
- Softened butter around 4 tablespoons
- Two Eggs
- Vanilla 1 teaspoon
- 3 tbsp. fresh cocoa butter melted
- 1/4 cup of almond flour
- 1 tablespoon of coconut flour
- 1/2 cup sweetener
- 1/4 cup of fresh cocoa butter diced

Directions

1. Preheat the baking oven to 350. Use cooking spray to cover the base of a 9 into 9 baking tray.

2. Beat the first 5 ingredients with an electric mixer until creamy. Bring the flour, sweetener, and sliced cocoa butter into the mixture. Scattered in a baking dish that has been prepared. Bake until the middle no longer jostles, and the corners are golden, for 25 minutes.

3. Cool thoroughly, and then, before slicing, chill in the freezer for 2-3 hours.

8. LOW CARB BAKED APPLES

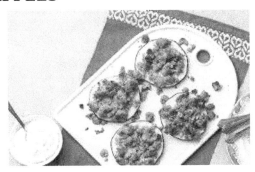

Serving: 4

Preparation time: 20 minutes

Nutritional values: 340kcal Calories | 88g Fat | 8g Carbs | 4g Proteins

Ingredients

- 2 ounces. cheese,
- 1 oz. Walnuts or Pecans
- 4 tablespoon coconut flour
- Cinnamon 1/2 tsp.
- Vanilla extract around 1/4 teaspoon
- One tart/sour apple

To serve

- 3/4 cup of heavy whipped cream
- Vanilla extract about 1/2 teaspoon

Directions

1. Heat the oven to 175°C (350°F). In a crispy dough, mix the hot butter, diced almonds, coconut flour, cinnamon & vanilla together.
2. Wash the apple, but don't eliminate the seeds or chop it. Cut both edges off and cut 4 slices through the center portion.
3. In a greased baking dish, put the slices and place dough crumbs on top. Bake fifteen minutes or more or until light brown appears on the crumbs.
4. To a moderate bowl, incorporate heavy whipping cream as well as vanilla and whisk until soft peaks appear.
5. For a minute or two, let the apples chilled and serve with a spoonful of whipped cream.

9. FROZEN YOGURT POPSICLES

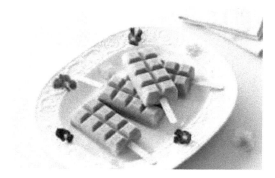

Serving: 12

Preparation time: 10mins 2hours

Nutritional values: 73kcal Calories | 60g Fat | 28g Carbs | 13g Proteins

Ingredients

- 8 oz. Mango chilled, chopped
- 8 oz. Strawberries chilled
- 1 cup of Greek full-fat yogurt
- 1/2 cup of heavy whipped cream
- 1 teaspoon extract of vanilla

Directions

1. Let the strawberries and mango defrost for 10 to 15 minutes.
2. In a mixer, place all the materials and combine until creamy.
3. End up serving as fluffy ice cream instantly or pipe into Popsicle shapes and chill for at least a few hours. If you do have an ice cream machine, it can be used, of course.

10. CHOCOLATE AVOCADO TRUFFLES

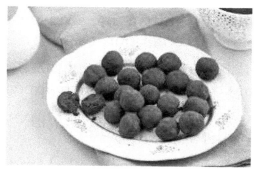

Serving: 20

Preparation time: 35 minutes

Nutritional values: 65kcal Calories | 76g Fat | 19g Carbs | 5g Proteins

Ingredients

- 1 (7 ounces.) ripe, diced avocado
- Vanilla extract about 1/2 teaspoon
- 1/2 lemon, zest
- About 1 pinch of salt
- Five ounces. Dark chocolate containing cocoa solids of at least 80 percent, finely diced
- 1 spoonful of coconut oil
- 1 tbsp. cocoa powder unsweetened

Directions

1. Use an electric mixer to mix the avocado and vanilla extract. The use of ripe avocado is necessary in order for the mixture to be fully creamy.
2. Add a tablespoon of salt and mix in the lemon zest.
3. In boiling water or oven, melt the chocolate & coconut oil.
4. Incorporate the chocolate & avocado and blend properly. Let it rest for 30 minutes in the fridge or until the batter is compact but not fully solid.
5. With your fingertips, shape little truffle balls. Likewise, use two teaspoons or a tiny scoop. Morph and roll in the cocoa powder with the hands.

11. CRUNCHY KETO BERRY MOUSSE

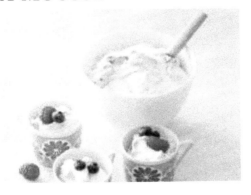

Serving: 8

Preparation time: 10 minutes

Nutritional values: 256kcal Calories | 26g Fat | 3g Carbs | 2g Proteins

Ingredients

- Two cups of heavy whipped cream
- Three ounces. Fresh strawberries or blueberries or raspberries
- 2 oz. Pecans diced
- 1/2 of a lime, zest
- Vanilla extract around 1/4 teaspoon

Directions

1. Drop the cream into a container and whip until soft peaks appear using a hand mixer. Towards the top, add the lime zest, then vanilla.
2. Cover the whipped cream with berries & nuts and stir thoroughly.
3. Wrap with plastic and allow for 3 or even more hours for a stable mousse to settle in the fridge. While you don't like a less firm consistency, you can also experience the dessert instantly.

Conclusion

Ketogenic' is a name for a diet that is low-carb. The concept is for you to obtain more protein and fat calories and fewer carbs. You reduce much of the carbs, such as sugar, coffee, baked goods, and white bread that are easily digestible.

If you consume fewer than 50 g of carbs a day, the body can gradually run out of resources (blood sugar) that you can use instantly. Usually, this takes 3 or 4 days. Then you're going to start breaking down fat and protein for nutrition, which will help with weight loss. This is classified as ketosis.

A ketogenic diet plan intended to induce ketosis, disintegrate body fat into ketones and enable the body to perform on ketones instead of glucose to a great extent. Since samen is the ultimate aim of these diets, there are typically a lot of connections between the various forms of the ketogenic diet, especially in terms of being low in carbohydrates and high in dietary fat. A program that focuses on high-fat and low carbohydrates is the Ketogenic Diet, and it has many advantages.

It is necessary to remember that a short-term diet that emphasizes weight reduction rather than medical benefits is a ketogenic diet. To reduce weight, people use a keto diet more commonly, although it may help treat some medical problems, such as epilepsy, too. People with heart problems, some neurological disorders, and also acne can even be supported, although further research in those fields needs to be conducted.

The Healthy Keto Meal Prep Cookbook with Pictures

Bend the Rules to Lose Weight Tasting Tens of Easy-to-Prep Ketogenic Recipes On a Budget

By

Gianna Carter

Table of Contents

Introduction

Few aspects are as well known in nutrition research as the tremendous health advantages of low-carb and ketogenic diets. Not only can these diets increase the cholesterol, blood pressure and blood sugar, but they also reduce your appetite, promote weight control and decrease the triglycerides.

A ketogenic diet may be an interesting way to manage such disorders and could accelerate weight loss. Yet it is challenging to follow, because it may be high on red meat and other oily, dried, and salty foods that are notoriously unhealthy. We still may not know anything about the long-term consequences, presumably because it's too hard to stay with that people can't eat this way for a long time. It is also important to note that "yo-yo diets" that contribute to rapid weight loss fluctuation are correlated with increased mortality. Instead of joining in the next common diet that will last just a few weeks or months (for most people that requires a ketogenic diet), strive to accept progress that is manageable over the long term. A healthy, unprocessed diet, abundant in very colorful fruits and vegetables, lean meats, seafood, whole grains, almonds, peas, olive oil, and plenty of water seems to provide the strongest evidence for a long, healthier, vibrant existence.

If you're interested to improve your fitness, this diet book might be worth considering.

Chapter 1: Keto Diet

The ketogenic (keto) diet is commonly known for having a diet (low crab), where the body creates ketones in the liver to be used as energy. It's alluded to by several different names – ketogenic diet, low carb diet, low carb high fat (LCHF), etc. When you consume something rich in carbohydrates, the body can release glucose and insulin.

Glucose is the simplest molecule for the body to transform and use as energy such that it can be preferred over some other energy source.

Insulin is created to process the glucose in your bloodstream by taking it across the body.

The glucose is being used as primary energy; the fats are not required and are thus processed. Usually, on a regular, higher carbohydrate diet, the body can use glucose as the key energy source. By lowering the consumption of carbohydrates, the body is induced into a condition known as ketosis. Ketosis, a normal mechanism the body initiates to help us live while food consumption is limited. During this state, we create ketones, which are formed by the oxidation of fats in the liver.

The ultimate aim of a well-controlled keto diet is to push your body into this physiological condition. We don't do this by deprivation of calories or starvation of carbohydrates.

What Do I Eat on a Keto Diet?

To initiate a keto diet, you may want to prepare accordingly. That implies getting a viable diet plan ready a. What you consume depends on how quickly you choose to get into a ketogenic condition, i.e., ketosis. The further stringent you are on your carbohydrates (less than 25g net carbs a day), the sooner you can reach ketosis.

You want to keep your carbs limited, come more from fruits, nuts, and dairy. Don't consume some processed grains such as wheat (bread, pasta, and cereals), starch (potatoes, beans, legumes) or berries. The small exceptions to this are banana, star fruit, and berries which may be eaten in moderation.

Do Not Eat

Grains: grain, maize, cereal, rice, etc.

Sugar: honey, maple syrup, agave, etc.

Fruit: bananas, grapes, strawberries, etc.

Tubers: yams, potatoes, etc.

Do Eat

Meats: fish, meat, lamb, chickens, chickens, etc.

Leafy Greens: lettuce, cabbage, etc.

Vegetables: broccoli, cauliflower, etc.

Low Fat Dairy: strong cheeses, high-fat milk, butter, etc.

Nuts and seeds: macadamias, walnuts, sunflower seeds, etc.

Avocado and berries – raspberries, blackberries, and other low glycemic

Sweeteners: stevia, erythritol, monk berries, and other low-carb sweeteners

Other fats: palm oil, high-fat salad dressing, fatty fats, etc.

Benefits of a Ketogenic Diet

Several advantages come from being on keto: from weight reduction and improved energy levels to medicinal uses. Mostly, everyone can easily profit from consuming a low-carb, high-fat diet. Below, you'll find a concise list of the advantages you may get from a ketogenic diet.

Weight Loss

The ketogenic diet actually utilizes your body fat as an energy source – but there are clear weight-loss advantages. On keto, your insulin (the fat-storing hormone) level drops greatly and transforms your body into a fat-burning process. Scientifically, the ketogenic diet has demonstrated better outcomes relative to low-fat and high-carb diets, also in the long run.

Control Blood Sugar

Keto reduces blood sugar levels due to the kinds of diet you consume. Studies also suggest that the ketogenic diet is a more efficient way to treat and avoid diabetes relative to low-calorie diets.

If you're pre-diabetic or have Type II diabetes, you should strongly try a ketogenic diet. We have several readers who have had experience in their blood sugar management on keto.

Mental Focus

Many people use the ketogenic diet primarily for improved mental output. Ketones are a perfect source of food for the brain. When you reduce carb consumption, you stop major increases in blood sugar. Together, which will help in increased attention and concentration? Studies suggest that an improved consumption of fatty acids may have affecting benefits to our brain's function.

Increased Energy & Normalized Hunger

By providing your body a stronger and more stable energy supply, you can feel more energized throughout the day. Fats are the most powerful molecule to burn as heat. On top of that, fat is inherently more rewarding and ends up keeping us in a satiated ("full") condition for longer.

Types of Ketogenic Diets

Many people wonder whether carbs are required to grow muscle. Actually, they're not. If you're asking this question, I will presume you know how you accumulate mass.

Your glycogen reserves will also be refilled while on a ketogenic diet. A keto diet is an effective way to grow muscle, but protein consumption is essential here. It's proposed that if you are trying to grow muscle, you could be getting in between 1.0 – 1.2g protein per lean pound of body mass. Putting muscle on can be slower on a ketogenic diet, but that's because the overall body fat is not growing as much.

If, for any reason, you need to add on body fat, too, you will accomplish your targets by various forms of a Ketogenic Diet. There are:

Standard Ketogenic Diet (SKD): This is the classic keto diet that everybody understands and does.

Targeted Ketogenic Diet (TKD): This variant is where you consume SKD but ingest a limited amount of fast-digesting carbohydrates before a workout.

Cyclical Ketogenic Diet (CKD): This variant of keto for bodybuilders and contests goers, usually offering one day a week to carb up and resupplies glycogen stocks.

Common Side Effects of a Keto Diet

Here are some of the more popular side effects that one comes across when people first initiate keto. Frequently the problems contribute to dehydration or loss of micronutrients (vitamins) in the body. Be sure that you're consuming enough water (close to a gallon a day) and enjoying foods containing healthy sources of micronutrients.

Cramps

Cramps (and, more importantly, leg cramps) are a fairly normal occurrence before beginning a ketogenic diet. It's typically happening in the morning or at night, but overall, it's a fairly small concern. It's a warning that there's a shortage of minerals, especially magnesium, in the body. Be sure you consume lots of fluid and eat salt on your meal. Using so will help reduce the lack of magnesium and get rid of the problem.

Constipation

The most frequent source of constipation is dehydration. An easy approach is to maximize water consumption and aim to get as close to a gallon a day as possible.

Trying to make sure veggies have some fiber. Bringing in some high-quality fiber from non-starchy vegetables will fix this issue. Though if that's not enough, normally, psyllium husk powder can work or take a probiotic.

Heart Palpitations

When switching to keto, you may find that the heart is beating both faster and slower. It's fairly normal, so don't think about it. If the condition remains, make sure that you're consuming enough liquids and eating enough salt. Usually, this is adequate to get rid of the issue right away. Though if the problem continues, it might be worth having a potassium supplement once a day.

Reduced Physical Performance

You can have some restrictions on your results when you start a keto diet, but it's generally only from your body transitioning to using fat, when your body changes in utilizing fat for energy, all of your power and stamina will return to normal. If you still notice issues with results, you can see benefits from taking carbs before exercising (or cycling carbs).

Saving Money and Budgeting

A popular myth is that the ketogenic diet is more costly than most diets out there. And, though it can be a little bit more costly than eating grain-stuffed goods, it's still better than many people believe. A ketogenic diet can be more costly than a regular American diet, but it's no different than most clean eating lifestyles. That said, there are always several ways to save money when cooking keto. The key strategies to raise money are the same as in all other budgeting:

Look for offers. There's still a discount or an offer to be had on keto-friendly products out there. Usually, you can find substantial discounts in magazines and newspapers that are delivered to your home, but they can also be paired with in-store specials and manager cuts. As paired, you will save a large portion of your keto groceries.

Bulk purchase and cook. If you're somebody who doesn't want to invest a lot of time in the kitchen, this is the best in all worlds. Buying the food at volume (specifically from wholesalers) will reduce the cost per pound immensely. Plus, you can make ahead food (bulk cook chicken thighs for pre-made beef, or cook whole meals) that are used as leftovers, meaning you waste less time preparing.

Do stuff yourself. Although it's incredibly easy to purchase certain products pre-made or pre-cooked, it still contributes to the price per pound of goods. Try prepping vegetables ahead of time instead of getting pre-cut ones. Try having your stew meat from a chuck roast. Or attempt to produce your mayo and salad dressings at home. The easiest of items will operate to cut back on your overall food shopping.

How to Reach Ketosis

Achieving ketosis is fairly simple, but it may appear complex and overwhelming for all of the details out there. Here's the bottom line about what you need to do, arranged in stages of importance:

Restrict the sugars: Many people prefer to only rely only on net carbohydrates. If you want better outcomes, restrict both. Aim to remain below 20g net carbs and below 35g gross carbs a day.

Restrict the protein consumption: Some people come over to keto from an Atkins diet and don't restrict their protein. Too much protein can contribute to lower levels of ketosis. Ideally, you ought to eat between 0.6g and 0.8g protein per pound of lean body fat. To assist with this, try using the keto calculator >

Stop thinking about fat: Fat is the main source of calories on keto – just be sure you're giving the body plenty of it. You should not lose weight on keto by malnutrition.

Drink water: Aim to drink a gallon of water a day. Make sure that you're hydrating and remaining compliant with the volume of water you consume. It not only helps regulate many important bodily functions, but it also helps manage hunger levels.

Stop snacking: Weight reduction seems to perform well because you have fewer insulin surges during the day. Unnecessary snacking can lead to stalls or delays in development.

Start fasting: Fasting can be a perfect tool to raise ketone levels reliably during the day. There are several different ways to go about it. Add workout in. It's a proven reality that exercise is safer. If you want to get the best out of your ketogenic diet, try putting in 20-30 minutes of workout a day. Also, only a short stroll will help control weight loss and blood sugar levels.

Begin supplementing: Although not normally required, supplementing can aid with a ketogenic diet.

What the Science Tell Us about the Keto Diet

The keto diet has been used to better treat epilepsy, a condition marked by seizures, for more than 100 years. More current trials are investigating the keto diet as an effective nutritional therapy for obesity and diabetes. Clinical results on the effects of the keto diet on these health problems are exceedingly minimal. Studies on the success of the keto diet are performed with limited groups of participants. And, much of the research on Alzheimer's disease depends on testing conducted on experimental animals. To completely evaluate the protection of this eating style, further study is required. Plus, research must be performed on the long-term health implications of the keto diet. Body mass index and human metabolic rates affect how easily various people generate ketones. This suggests that certain individuals lose weight more slowly with the keto diet than others even though they are pursuing the same keto diet schedule. For this community of individuals, the keto diet may be stressful and can affect their enthusiasm for making healthy lifestyle improvements. Plus, many individuals are not willing to continue with the keto diet and gain back weight after adjusting to their former eating style.

Chapter 2: Keto Diet Breakfast Recipes

Keto Hot Chocolate

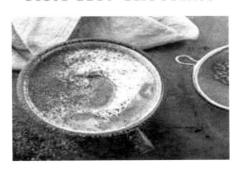

YIELDS: 1

TOTAL TIME: 0 HOURS **20** MINS.

INGREDIENTS

- • 2 Tbsp. of cocoa powder, and more for flavor
- • 2 1/2 Tsp. of sugar keto (diet), (such as swerve)
- • 1 1/4 c. of Water
- • 1/4 c. of heavy cream
- • 1/4 Tsp. of Pure vanilla bean paste
- • Whipped serum, for serving

DIRECTIONS

1. In a small saucepan over medium-low heat, whisk together swerve, cocoa powder or about 2 Tbs. water until smooth and dissolved. Increase heat to medium, add remaining water and cream, and whisk until cook.

2. Mix the chocolate then pour into cup. Serve with whipped cream and a dusting of sugar powder.

Keto Sausage Breakfast Sandwich

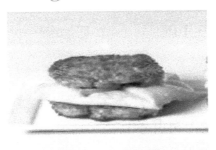

YIELDS: 3

TOTAL TIME: 0 HOURS 15 MINS

INGREDIENTS

- 6 large size eggs

- 2 Tbsp. of heavy cream
- Pinch of red chili flakes
- Salt (kosher)
- Finely roasted black pepper
- 1 Tbsp. of butter
- 3 slices of cheddar
- 6 packaged of sausage burgers, cooked as per box directions
- Avocado, sliced

DIRECTIONS

1. Take a small bowl beat eggs, red chili flakes and heavy cream jointly. Season with pepper and salt. Melt the butter in fry pan at low flame. Add around one third of eggs in to pan. Add a piece of cheese in the center or let stay for 1 minute. Roll the ends of egg in to center, filling a cheese. Take out from heat and continue with leftover egg.

2. Serve eggs in 2 sausage buns with avocado.

Keto Breakfast Cups

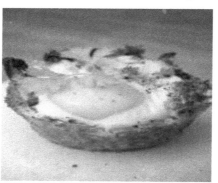

YIELDS: 12

TOTAL TIME: 0 HOURS **40** MINS

INGREDIENTS

- 2 Ib. of Pork (ground)
- 1 Tbsp. thyme, finely sliced
- 2 cloves of garlic, finely chopped
- 1/2 Tsp. of Paprika
- 1/2 Tsp. of cumin, ground
- 1 Tsp. of Salt kosher
- Black pepper softly roasted
- 21/2 cup of clean minced spinach
- 1 c. of cheddar, thinly sliced
- Eggs, 12
- 1 Tbsp. of chives that are finely cut

DIRECTIONS

1. 1 Preheat the oven at 400 degrees. Combine the thyme, ground pork, paprika, garlic, salt, and cumin in a large size cup.

2. In each muffin container, add a tiny handful of pork and push up the sides to make a cup. Split the cheese and spinach equally in cups. Break the egg and add the salt and pepper on the top of each cup. Cook for around 25 minutes until the eggs are fixed and the sausage is fried.
3. Garnish and serve with chives.

Best-Ever Cabbage Hash Browns

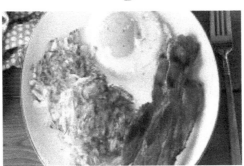

YIELDS: 2

TOTAL TIME: 0 HOURS **25** MINS

INGREDIENTS

- 2 Large size eggs
- 1/2 Tsp. of garlic, powdered
- 1/2 Tsp. of salt (kosher)
- Freshly roasted black pepper
- 2c. of cabbage that is shredded
- ¼ of small size yellow onions, finely chopped
- 1 Tbsp. of oil (vegetable)

DIRECTIONS

1. Whisk the garlic powder, salt, and eggs together in a large cup. Add black pepper for seasoning. In egg mixture add onion and cabbage and toss to mix properly.
2. Heat oil in a large frying pan. Split the mixture in the pan into 4 patties and press spatula to soften. Cook until soft and golden, around three minutes on each side.

Chocolate Keto Protein Shake

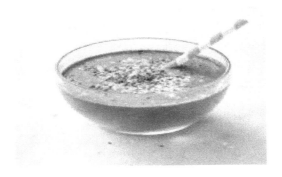

YIELD: 1
TOTAL TIME: 0 HOURS 5 MINS
INGREDIENTS

- 3/4 c of almond milk
- 1/2 c. of ice
- 2 Tbsp. of Butter (almond)
- 2 Tbsp. of (Sugar free) powder of cocoa
- 3 Tbsp. of keto-diet sugar substitute as per taste (such as Swerve)
- 1Tbsp. seeds of chia or more for serving
- 2 Tbsp. seeds of hemp, or more for serving
- 1/2 Tbsp. of pure vanilla (extracted)
- Salt kosher as per taste

DIRECTIONS

1. Merge all of blending mixture and mix untill soft. Put into glass and serve with hemp seed and chia.

Hard Boiled Egg

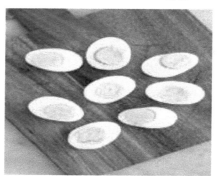

YIELDS: 1
TOTAL TIME: 0 HOURS 20 MINS
INGREDIENTS

- 12 large size eggs
- Some water

DIRECTIONS

1. Place the eggs in such a wide saucepan and cover them with one inch of ice water. Keep the saucepan on the burner and get it to a boil. Immediately turn off the flame and cover the saucepan. Let settle down for eleven minutes.
2. Take it out from the pan and switch it to ice water. Until serving or peeling, let it cool for 2 minutes.

Paleo Breakfast Stacks

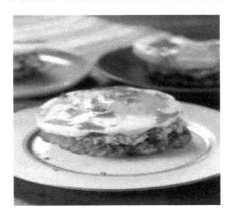

YIELDS: 3

TOTAL TIME: 0 HOURS 30 MINS

INGREDIENTS

- 3 sausage buns for breakfast
- 1 avocado, finely mashed
- Salt (kosher)
- Black pepper freshly roasted
- 3 large size eggs
- Chives, (for serving)
- Hot sauce, if ordered

DIRECTIONS

1. Cook the breakfast sausage as per the box's instructions.
2. Mash the avocado over the sausage for breakfast and season with pepper and salt.
3. Use cooking oil to spray the medium size pan then spray the interior of mason jar cover. Place the mason jar lid in the middle of the pan and crack the interior of an egg. Add pepper or salt and cook until the whites are set for 3 minutes, then remove the cover and begin to cook.
4. Place the egg on top of the avocado puree. Serve with chives and drizzle with your favorite spicy hot sauce.

Ham & Cheese Breakfast Roll-Ups

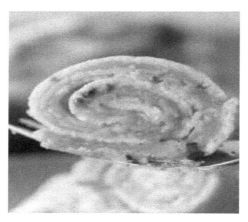

YIELDS: 2

TOTAL TIME: 0 HOURS **20** MINS

INGREDIENT

- 4 large size eggs
- 1/4 c of milk
- 2 Tbsp. of finely cut chives
- Salt (kosher)
- Black pepper freshly roasted
- 1Tbsp. of butter
- 1c. of cheddar shredded,(Split)
- 4 slices of ham

DIRECTIONS

1. Whisk the milk, chives, and egg together in a medium cup. Add pepper or salt.
2. Melt the butter in a medium pan over low heat. Put 1/2 of the egg mixture in the pan and shift to make a thin layer that covers the whole plan.
3. Cook for two minutes. Add1/2 cup of cheddar or seal again for 2 minutes, before the cheese has melted transfer to plate, and put 2 slices of ham or rolls them. Repeat and cook with the rest of the ingredients.

Cauliflower Toast

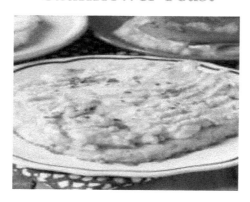

YIELDS: 4 - 6

TOTAL TIME: 0 HOURS **45** MINS

INGREDIENTS

- 1 cauliflower (in medium size)
- Large size egg
- 1/2 c. of cheddar cheese (shredded)
- 1Tsp.of garlic(powdered)
- Salt (kosher)
- Black pepper freshly roasted

DIRECTIONS

1. Set the oven at 425 degree temperature and cover the baking sheet with parchment paper. Finely chopped the cauliflower and   switch to a large size cup. Set the microwave at high temperature for 8 minutes. Drain with cheesecloth and paper towels just before the mixture is dry.
2. In cauliflower cup, add the cheddar, garlic powder and egg and season with pepper and salt. Mix it until joint
3. Make a cauliflower into bread forms on prepared baking sheet and bake for 18 to 20 minutes until golden.
4. Switch to a plate cover with the appropriate topping, such as fried egg, mashed avocado, tomato, broccoli, and sausage.

Breakfast Bacon and Egg Salad

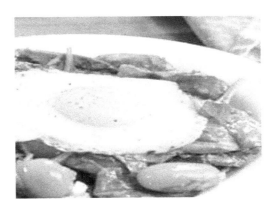

YIELDS: 4

TOTAL TIME: 0 HOURS **30** MINS

INGREDIENTS

Bacon vinaigrette

- 4 bacon (slices)
- 1 shallot, thinly sliced
- 3 Tbsp. of red wine(vinegar)
- 1 Tsp. of mustard (Dijon)
- 1/4 Tsp. of salt (kosher)
- 1/4 Tsp. of black pepper
- 4 Tbsp. of Oil

Salad

2   small size eggs
1 Spinach (package)
1/4 c. of crumbled feta
1 pt. of tomatoes and cherry

DIRECTIONS

1. In a large fry pan, cook the bacon. Remove the bacon slices and put on a plate and line with towel paper to drain. Implode half of the bacon until the excess fat has drained, then cut the rest of two pieces into large pieces. Set again.

2. Making the vinaigrette: Add the shallot into the pot in which the bacon has been fried, and sauté for around 1 minute over moderate flame until golden brown. Pour the shallots into a small cup and blend with the pepper, salt, red vinegar, and mustard. Whisk in the oil, and then add the crumbled bacon and blending to combine. Set again.

3. In the same pot, fried each egg and cook until the egg white is fixed.
4. Assemble the salad: Combine the feta, lettuce, tomatoes, cherry, spinach and the remaining sliced bacon in a large size dish. Cover with vinaigrette.
5. Place the salad in two cups and cover it with the fried egg. Immediately serve.

Keto Blueberry Muffins

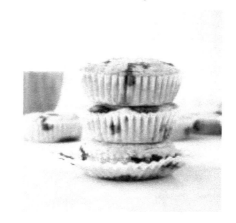

YIELD: 1

TOTAL TIME: 0 HOURS **40** MINS

INGREDIENTS

- 2 1/2 c. of almond Flour

- 1/3 c. of Keto diet sugar (such as Swerve)

- 1 1/2 Tsp. of baking powder

- 1/2 Tsp. of baking soda

- 1/2 Tsp. salt kosher

- 1/3 c. of melted butter

- 1/3 c. of Sugar free almonds milk

- 3 large size eggs
- 1 Tsp. of pure vanilla extract
- 2/3 of c. of fresh blueberries
- ½ of lemon zest (as an option)

DIRECTIONS

1. Preheat oven to 350° and line a 12-cup muffin pan with cupcake liners.
2. In a large bowl, whisk to combine baking powder, baking soda, almond flour, salt kosher and swerve. Whisk in eggs, vanilla, almond milk, melted butter and almond milk until just together.
3. Gently fold lemon zest (if using) and blueberries until uniformly divided. Scoop uniform quantity of butter into every cupcake liner and cook until slightly golden brown and insert a toothpick into the middle of a muffin comes out clean, 23 minutes. Let cool slightly before presenting.

Mason Jar Omelets

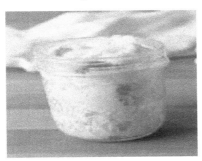

YIELDS: 2

TOTAL TIME: 0 HOURS 15 MINS

INGREDIENTS

- Nonstick cooking oil
- 4 large size eggs
- 2/3 c. of cheddar shredded
- ½ of onion, thinly sliced
- 1 Chopped capsicum
- 1/2 c. of ham (sliced)
- Salt kosher
- Freshly roasted black pepper
- 1Tbsp. of Chives that are finely sliced

DIRECTIONS

1. Oil the nonstick baking spray into two liter mason jars.
2. Break two eggs into each jar. Between two jar divide the onion, ham capsicum, and cheese and season with pepper and salt.
3. Put cover on jar and mix until eggs are scrambled and all ingredients are mixed.
4. Remove the cover and place in the oven. Microwave for 4 minutes on low flame, and looking every 30 seconds. Garnish with chives, and serve immediately.

Keto Fat Bombs

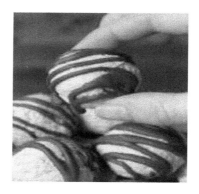

YIELDS: 16

TOTAL TIME: 0 HOURS **30** MIN

INGREDIENTS

- 8 oz. of cream cheese, mitigated at room temp.
- 1/2 c. of keto diet (peanuts) butter
- 1/4 c of (coconut oil)
- 1/4 Tsp. of salt (kosher)
- 1/2 c. of dark chocolate (keto diet) (such as Lily's)

DIRECTIONS

1. Cover the baking sheet with a tiny parchment paper. Mix the peanut butter, salt, cream cheese and 1/4 cup of coconut oil in a medium dish. With the help of hand blender beat the mixture for around 2 minutes until all ingredients are properly mixed. Keep the dish for 10 to 15 minutes in the freezer to firm up slightly.
2. Using a tiny cookie spoon or scoop to make a Tbs. sized balls until the (peanut butter) mixture has been settled. Keep in the freezer for 5 minutes to harden.
3. Besides that, making a drizzle of chocolate: mix the cocoa powder and the leftover coconut oil in a safe microwave dish and cook for 30 seconds until completely melt. Drizzle over the balls of peanut butter and put them back in the fridge to harden for 5 minutes.
4. Keep the cover and freeze it for storage purpose.

Cloud Eggs

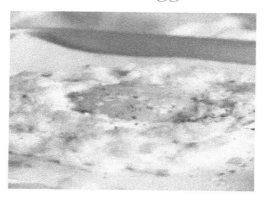

YIELDS: 4

TOTAL TIME: 0 HOURS **20** MINS

INGREDIENTS

- 8 large size eggs
- 1 c. of Parmesan, thinly sliced
- 1/2 lb. of Ham deli, diced
- Salt (kosher)
- Freshly made black pepper
- For serving, finely sliced chives

DIRECTIONS

1. Heat the oven at 450 °C and spread cooking oil on a large baking sheet. Separate the yolks and egg whites, yolks are keep in small cup and egg whites are keep in large cup egg whites. Use a hand blender or whisk break egg whites before stiff peaks shape and cook for 3 minutes. Fold in the ham and parmesan or season with pepper and salt.
2. Spoon the 8 mounds of egg onto the heated baking dish and indent centers to make nests. Cook for around 3 minutes, until lightly golden.
3. Spoon the egg yolk cautiously into the middle of each nest, then season with pepper or salt. Cook for around 3 minutes more until the yolks are ready.
4. Before presenting, garnish it with chives.

Chapter 3: Keto Diet Lunch Recipes

Cobb Egg Salad

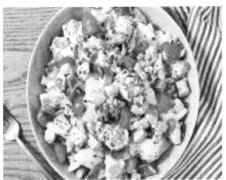

YIELDS: 6

TOTAL TIME: 0 HOURS **20** MINS

INGREDIENTS

- 3 Tbsp. of mayonnaise
- 3 Tbsp. of yogurt
- 2 tbsp. of vinegar with red wine
- Salt (kosher)
- Black pepper freshly roasted
- 8 hard-boiled eggs, sliced into 8 pieces, and more for garnishing.
- 8 bacon strips, fried and crumbled, and more for garnishing.
- 1 avocado, cut finely
- 1/2 c. of blue cheese, crumbled, and more for garnishing
- 1/2 c. of halved cherry tomatoes, and more for garnishing
- 2 Tbsp. of chives that are finely chopped

DIRECTIONS

1. Mix the yogurt, red vinegar and mayonnaise together in a small cup. Seasoning with pepper and salt.
2. Mix the avocado, bacon, eggs, pineapple, cherry tomatoes and blue cheese, softly together in a large serving cup. Gently roll in the mayonnaise coating until the all ingredients are finely coated, and then sprinkle with pepper and salt.
3. Serving with chives and supplementary toppings

Taco Stuffed Avocado

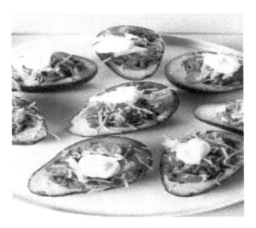

YIELDS: 4 - 8

TOTAL TIME: 0 HOURS 25 MINS

INGREDIENTS

- 4 large size avocados
- 1 lime juice
- 1 Tbsp. of olive oil (extra-virgin)
- 1 medium size onion, minced
- 1 lb. minced meat of beef
- 1 taco seasoning pack
- Salt (kosher)
- Blinerack pepper freshly roasted
- 2/3 of c. of chopped Mexican cheese
- 1/2 c. of chopped Lettuce
- 1/2 c. of Grape tomatoes (Sliced)
- Sour milk, for garnishing

DIRECTIONS

1. Pit and halve the avocados halve and pit. Scoop out a bit of avocado with the help of a spoon, forming a wide layer. Dice extracted avocado and later put aside for use. Pinch the lime juice (to avoid frying!) at all the avocados.
2. Heat the oil in a medium size pan over medium heat. Add the onion and roast for around 5 minutes, until soft. Break up the meat with a wooden spatula then add ground beef and taco for seasoning. Sprinkle with pepper and salt, and roast for around 6 minutes until the beef is no more pink. Drain the fat after removing from the heat.
3. Fill up the each avocado halve with meat, then and coat with cheese, reserved avocado, tomato, onion, lettuce, and a dollop of sour cream.

Buffalo Shrimp Lettuce Wraps

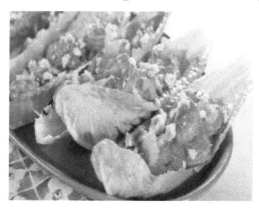

YIELDS: 4

TOTAL TIME: 0 HOURS **35** MINS

INGREDIENTS

- 1/4 Tbsp. of butter
- 2 cloves of garlic, chopped
- 1/4 c. of Hot sauce, for example, Frank's
- 1 Tbsp. of olive oil (extra-virgin)
- 1 lbs. of Chopped and finely diced shrimp, tails (cut)
- Salt kosher
- Black pepper freshly roasted
- 1 head Romaine, different leaves, for garnishing
- 1/4 of red onion, finely minced
- 1 rib celery, finely chopped
- 1/2 c. of Crumbled blue cheese

DIRECTIONS

1. Making the buffalo sauce: Melt the butter in a small pan. When fully melted, then add chopped garlic and simmer for 1 minute, until golden brown. Add hot sauce and stir together. Switch the heat to low whilst the shrimp is frying.
2. Making shrimp: Heat oil in a large frying pan. Put some shrimp and sprinkle with pepper and salt. Cook, turning midway, until both sides are opaque and pink, around 2 minutes on each side. Turn off the flame and add the (buffalo) sauce and toss to fill.
3. Prepare wraps: In the middle of the romaine leaf add a little scoop of shrimp, then coat with celery, blue cheese and red onion.

Keto Broccoli Salad

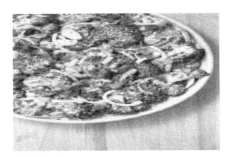

YIELDS: 4
TOTAL TIME: 0 HOURS **35** MINS
INGREDIENTS

For the salad:

- Salt (kosher)
- 3 broccoli heads, sliced into bite-size parts
- 1/2 c. of cheddar shredded
- 1/4 red onion, finely cut
- 1/4 c. of almonds sliced (baked)
- 3 bacon slices, fried and crumbled
- 2 Tbsp. of Chives that are finely cut

For the dressing:

- 2/3 of c. of mayonnaise
- 3 Tbsp. of Vinegar (Apple Cider)
- 1 Tbsp. of Mustard dijon
- salt kosher
- Black pepper freshly roasted

DIRECTIONS

1. Bring the 6 cups of (salted) water to a boil in a medium pot or frying pan. Prepare a big bowl of ice water while waiting for the water to heat.
2. Put some broccoli florets to the boiling water and simmer for 1 to 2 minutes, until soft. Detach with a slotted spoon, and put in the prepared ice water cup. Drain the florets in a colander while it is cold.
3. In a medium dish, whisk together the ingredients for the dressing. Season with pepper and salt to taste.
4. In a large bowl, combine all the salad ingredients and pour over the coating. Toss before the components are coated in the dressing. Refrigerate until prepared

Keto Bacon Sushi

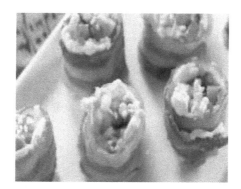

YIELDS: 12

TOTAL TIME: 0 HOURS **30** MINS

INGREDIENTS

- 6 bacon pieces, (halved)
- 2 Persian cucumbers, cut finely
- 2 medium size carrots, cut finely
- 1 avocado, in slices
- 4 oz. of melted cream cheese, (cooked)

DIRECTIONS

1. Preheat oven to 400 ° degrees. Cover a baking sheet and match it with a cooling rack and aluminum foil. Put some bacon pieces in an even layer and cook for 11 to 13 minutes until mildly crisp but still pliable.
2. Mean a while, cut avocado, cucumbers, and broccoli into pieces around the width of bacon.
3. Spread an equal layer of cream cheese on each slice until the bacon is cold enough to touch it. Split up the vegetables between the bacon uniformly and put them on one side. Tightly roll up the vegetables.
4. Serve and garnish with sesame seeds.

Keto Burger Fat Bombs

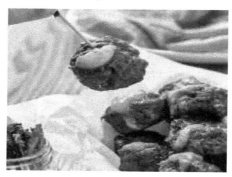

YIELDS: 20

TOTAL TIME: 0 HOURS **30** MINS

INGREDIENTS

- Cooking oil
- 1 lbs. of ground-based meat
- 1/2 Tsp. of Powdered garlic
- Salt Kosher
- Black pepper freshly roasted
- 2 Tbsp. of cold butter,20 (sliced)
- 2 oz. of cheddar cheese 20 (sliced)
- Lettuce berries, meant for garnishing
- For garnishing, finely sliced tomatoes
- Mustard, for garnishing

DIRECTIONS

1. Preheat the oven at 375 °C and oil mini muffin container with cooking oil. And season the beef with garlic powder, salt, and pepper in a medium dish.
2. In the bottom of each muffin tin cup add the 1 Tsp. of beef equally, and fully covering the bottom. Place a layer of butter on top and add 1 Tsp. of beef over the butter to fully cover.
3. In each cup, place a slice of cheddar on top of the meat and place the remaining beef over the cheese to fully cover.
4. Bake for about 15 minutes, before the meat is ready. Let wait until cool.
5. Using a metal offset spoon carefully to release each burger out of the tin. Serve with salad leaves, mustard and onions.

Keto Taco Cups

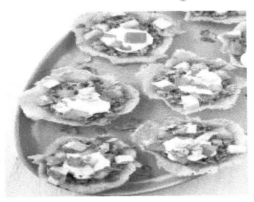

YIELDS: 1 DOZEN

TOTAL TIME: 0 HOURS **30 MINS**

INGREDIENTS

- 2 c. of Cheddar (Sliced) cheese
- 1 Tbsp. of Olive Oil (extra-Virgin)
- 1 small size chopped onion
- 3 cloves of garlic , finely chopped
- 1 lbs. of meat, ground

- 1 Tsp. of chili(in powdered form)
- 1/2 Tsp. of Cumin ,ground
- 1/2 tsp. of Paprika
- Salt (kosher)
- Black pepper freshly roasted
- Sour cream, to serve
- Diced avocado, planned for serving
- Cilantro finely chopped, for serving
- Tomatoes, chopped, for garnishing

DIRECTIONS

1. Preheat the oven to 375 ° and use parchment paper to cover a wide baking sheet. Add 2 teaspoons of cheddar a half inch away. Cook for around 6 minutes, until creamy and the edges begin to turn golden. Leave the baking sheet for a minute until cool.
2. Besides that, apply the oil in the muffin tin bottom with a cooking spray, then carefully pick up the slices of melted cheese and put them on the muffin tin bottom. Add another inverted muffin container until cool for 10 minutes. Using your hands to help shape the cheese around the twisted pan because you do not have a second muffin tin.
3. Preheat the large size pan over medium heat. Put the onion and simmer for around 5 minutes, mixing frequently, until soft. Whisk in the garlic, then add the ground beef to break up the beef with the help of wooden spoon. Cook for around 6 minutes, until the beef is no longer pink, and then drain the fat.
4. Place the meat back in the pan and season with cumin, chili powder, cinnamon, paprika, and pepper.
5. Move the cups of cheese into a serving bowl. Cover it with cooked ground beef and serve with cilantro, sour cream, tomatoes, and avocado.

Copycat Chicken Lettuce Wraps

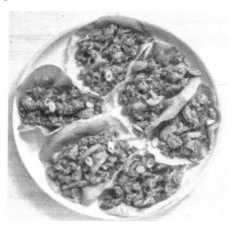

YIELDS: 4

TOTAL TIME: 0 HOURS **30** MINS

INGREDIENTS

- 3 Tbsp. of Sauce (Hoisin)
- 2 Tbsp. Soy sauce (low-sodium)
- 2 Tbsp. vinegar from rice wine
- 1 Tbsp. of sriracha (as an option)
- 1 Tsp. oil with sesame seeds
- 1 Tbsp. olive oil (extra-virgin)
- 1 medium size chopped onion
- 2 cloves of garlic, chopped
- 1 Tbsp. of freshly coated ginger
- 1 lbs. of Chicken, ground
- 1/2 c. of drained and diced canned water chestnuts
- 2 green onions, cut finely
- Salt kosher
- Black pepper freshly roasted
- Large leafy lettuce for serving (leaves separated),
- Fried white rice, for garnishing(as an option)

DIRECTIONS

1. Making a sauce: Whisk together the soya sauce, the hoisin sauce, the sriracha the rice wine vinegar, the Sriracha and the sesame oil in a tiny cup.
2. Heat the olive oil in a large pan over a medium-high heat. Put some onions and cook for 5 minutes until soft, then stir the garlic and ginger and cook for 1 more minute until golden brown. Add ground chicken and cook until the meat is opaque and mostly finished, trying to break up the meat with a wooden spoon.

3. Add the sauce and simmer again for 1 or 2 minutes, before the sauce is slightly reduced and the chicken is thoroughly cooked. Switch off the flame, add green onions and chestnuts and mix. Season with pepper and salt.
4. Spoon rice and add a big scoop of chicken mixture (about 1/4 cup) into the middle of each lettuce leaf (if used). Instantly serve

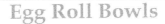

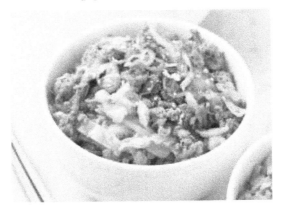

YIELDS: 4

TOTAL TIME: 0 HOURS 35 MINS

INGREDIENTS

- 1 Tbsp. of oil for vegetables
- 1 clove of garlic, chopped
- 1 Tbsp. fresh ginger chopped
- 1 lbs. of pork, ground
- 1 Tbsp. of oil with sesame seeds
- 1/2 onion, cut finely
- 1 c. of Carrot(sliced)
- 1/4 green, thinly sliced (cabbage)
- 1/4 c. of soya sauce
- 1 Tbsp. of sriracha
- 1 small size green onion, finely chopped
- 1 Tbsp. of sesame seeds

DIRECTIONS

1. Heat the vegetable oil in a large skillet over medium heat. Add the garlic and ginger and roast for 1 to 2 minutes until it is moist. Add pork and roast until there is no more pink color has been shown.
2. Place the pork and add the sesame oil to other side. Add the tomato, cabbage, and potato. Add the soy sauce and Sriracha and whisk to combine with the beef. Cook for 5 to 8 minutes, until the cabbage is soft.
3. Garnish with sesame seeds and green onions and shift the mixture to a serving bowl. Serve immediately.

Caprese Zoodles

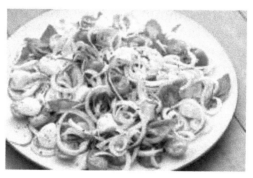

YIELDS: 4

TOTAL TIME: 0 HOURS **25** MINS

INGREDIENTS

- 4 large size zucchinis
- 2 Tbsp. of olive oil (extra-virgin)
- Kosher salt
- Black pepper freshly roasted
- 2 c. of cherry tomatoes, sliced in half
- 1 c. of mozzarella cubes, cut into pieces(if large)

- 1/4 c.   fresh leaves of basil
- 2 Tbsp. of vinegar (balsamic)
- DIRECTIONS
1. Using a spiralizer, make zoodles with the help of zucchini.
2. In a large cup, add the zoodles mix with the olive oil, and add pepper and salt. Let them marinate for 15 minutes.
3. Add the basil, peppers, and mozzarella in zoodles and toss until mixed.
4. Drizzle and serve with balsamic.

Best-Ever Keto Quesadillas

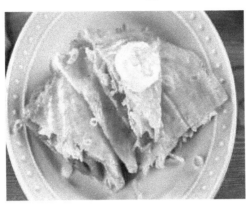

YIELDS: 4

TOTAL TIME: 0 HOURS 35 MINS

INGREDIENTS

- 1 Tbsp. of olive oil (extra-virgin)
- 1 chopped bell pepper
- 1/2 of onion(yellow), chopped
- 1/2 Tsp. of chili powdered
- Salt kosher
- Black pepper freshly roasted
- 3 c. of Monterey jack shredded
- 3 c. of cheddar cheese, shredded
- 4 c. of Chicken shredded
- 1 avocado, cut thinly
- 1 green onion, finely chopped
- Sour cream, for serving

DIRECTIONS

1. Preheat the oven to 400C and cover the parchment paper with two medium size baking sheets.
2. Heat the oil in a medium saucepan over medium heat. Season with salt, chili powder and pepper and add onion and pepper. Cook for 5 minutes, until it is tender. Transfer to a dish.

3. In a medium cup, mix the cheeses together. In the middle of both prepared baking sheets, add 1 1/2 cups of cheese mixture. Spread into an even coat and form the size of a flour tortilla into a circle.

4. Bake the cheeses for 8 to 10 minutes before they are melted and slightly golden along the sides. Add one half of avocado slices, onion-pepper mixture, shredded chicken and avocado slices. Let it cool slowly, then use the small spoon and parchment paper and carefully fold and lift one end of the cheese "tortilla" over the end with the topping. Return to the oven to heat for an extra 3 to 4 minutes. To make 2 more quesadillas, repeat the procedure.

5. Split each quesadilla into quarters. Before serving, garnish it with sour cream and green onion.

Cheeseburger Tomatoes

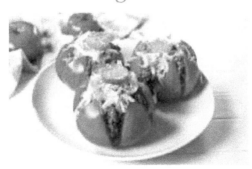

YIELDS: 4

TOTAL TIME: 0 HOURS **20** MINS

INGREDIENTS

- 1 Tbsp. of olive oil (extra-virgin)
- 1 medium size onion, minced
- 2 cloves of garlic, chopped
- 1 lbs. of ground-based meat
- 1 Tbsp. of ketchup
- 1 Tbsp. of mustard (Yellow)
- 4 sliced tomatoes
- Salt kosher
- Black paper freshly roasted
- 2/3 of c. of cheddar shredded
- 1/4 c. of Iceberg lettuce shredded
- 4 coins with pickles
- Seeds of sesame, for garnishing

DIRECTIONS

1. Heat oil in a medium pan over medium heat. Add the onion and cook for approximately 5 minutes until soft, then add the garlic. Add the ground beef, split up the meat with a wooden spoon and roast for around 6 minutes until the beef is no longer pink. Drain fats. Season with pepper and salt, then add the ketchup and mustard.

2. Because they are stem-side out, tossing tomatoes. Cut the tomatoes into six slices and be cautious not to cut the tomatoes full. Fold the slices carefully. Divide the tomatoes equally with the cooked ground beef, then fill it with lettuce and cheese.
3. Add sesame seeds and pickle coins for flavoring.

No-Bread Italian Subs

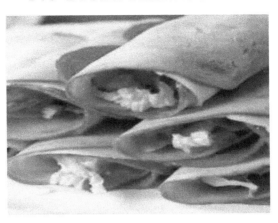

YIELDS: 6

TOTAL TIME: 0 HOURS **15** MINS

INGREDIENTS

- 1/2 c. of mayonnaise
- 2 Tbsp. of Vinegar with red wine
- 1 Tbsp. olive oil (extra-virgin)
- 1 tiny clove of garlic, finely chopped
- 1 Tsp. of seasoning (Italian)
- 6 slices of ham
- 12 salami sliced
- 12 pepperoni, sliced
- 6 provolone slices
- 1 c. of romaine(chopped)
- 1/2 c. of red peppers (roasted)

DIRECTIONS

1. Making a smooth Italian dressing: whisk the mustard, mayonnaise, garlic, oil, and Italian seasoning together in a small bowl until they are mixed.
2. Prepare the sandwiches: Layer a pieces of pork, two pieces of pepperoni, two pieces of salami and a piece of provolone.
3. In the center, add a handful of Romaine and a few roasted red peppers. Drizzle, with fluffy Italian sauce, then roll up and eat. Continue the procedure with the rest of the ingredients until you have 6 roll-ups.

California Burger Bowls

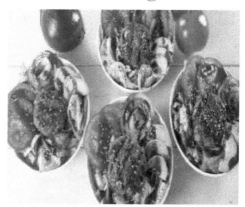

YIELDS: 4

TOTAL TIME: 0 HOURS **20** MINS

INGREDIENTS

For the dressing:

- 1/2 c. of olive oil (extra-virgin)
- 1/3 c. of vinegar (balsamic)
- 3Tbsp. of mustard dijon
- 2 Tsp. of. honey
- 1 clove of garlic , chopped
- Salt kosher
- Black pepper freshly roasted

For the burger:

- 1 lbs. of grass fed organic ground beef
- 1 Tsp. of Sauce (worcestershire)
- 1/2 tsp. of chili Powdered
- 1/2 tsp. onion Powdered
- Salt kosher
- Black pepper freshly roasted
- 1 packet of butter head lettuce
- 1 medium size red onion, sliced (¼)
- 1 avocado,(in pieces)
- 2 Walmart medium size tomato, thinly sliced

DIRECTIONS

1. Making the dressing: Whisk together the dressing components in a medium dish.
2. Making burgers: Mix beef with chili powder, (Worcestershire) sauce and onion powder in another large bowl. Season with salt and pepper and whisk until blend. Shape into 4 patties.
3. Heat a wide grill pan over medium heat and grill the onions until they are crispy and soft, around 3 minutes on at each end. Remove the grill from the pan and add

the burgers. Bake until browned and fried to your taste on all ends, around 4 minutes per end for medium.

4. Assemble: Toss the lettuce with 1/2 of the dressing in a wide bowl and split between 4 bowls. Cover each with a patty of steak, tomatoes, fried onions, slices of 1/4 avocado. Drizzle and serve with the remaining dressing.

Chapter 4: Dinner Recipes

Keto Corned Beef & Cabbage

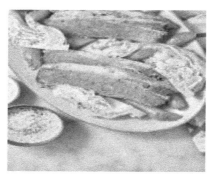

TOTAL TIME: 5 HOURS 0 MINS

YIELDS: 6

INGREDIENTS:

- 3 to 4 1bs. of corned beef
- Onions, 2 (quartered)
- 4 stalks of, quartered crosswise celery
- 1 pack of pickling spices
- Salt (Kosher)
- Black Pepper
- 1 medium size cabbage (green), sliced into 2 wedges
- carrots (2), sliced and split into 2" part
- 1/2 c. of Dijon mustard
- 2 Tbsp. of (apple cider) vinegar
- 1/4 c. of mayonnaise
- 2 Tbsp. capers, finely sliced, plus 1 tsp. of brine
- 2 Tbsp. of parsley, finely cut

Directions:

1. Place corned beef, onion, celery, and pickling spices into a large pot. Add the water to cover by 2", salt with season or Pepper, and bring to the boil. Medium heat, cover, and Simmer very (tender), 3–3 1/2 hours.
2. In the meantime, whisk Dijon mustard and apple cider vinegar in a small bowl and add salt and pepper. And in another bowl, mix capers, mayo, caper brine, and parsley. Season with salt and pepper
3. Added carrots and cabbage continue cooking for 45 minutes to 1 hour more until cabbage is soft. Remove meat, cabbage, and carrots from the pot. Piece of corned beef and season with a little more pepper and salt.
4. Present with both sauces on the side for soaking.

Keto Fried Chicken:

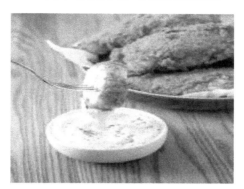

TOTAL TIME: 1 HOUR 15 MINS

YIELDS: 6 - 8

INGREDIENTS

FOR THE CHICKEN

- 6 (Bone-in), chicken breasts with skin, about 4 lbs.
- Salt (Kosher)
- Black Pepper, ground and fresh
- 2 large size eggs
- 1/2 c. of heavy cream
- 3/4 c. of almond flour
- 1 1/2 c. perfectly crushed pork rinds
- 1/2 c. of grated Parmesan, fresh
- 1 Tsp. of Garlic in powder form
- 1/2 Tsp. of paprika

FOR THE SPICY MAYO:

- 1/2 c. of Mayonnaise
- 1 1/2 Tsp. of Hot sauce

DIRECTIONS

1. Preheat oven to 400° and cover a wide baking sheet with parchment paper. Pat dry chicken with paper towels and add salt and pepper.
2. In a small bowl, mix together eggs and heavy cream. In another small dish, mix almond flour, pork rinds, Parmesan, garlic powder, and paprika. Add salt and black pepper.
3. Work at one time, soak the chicken in egg mix, then in the almonds flour mix, pressing to cover. Put the chicken on the lined baking dish.
4. Bake till chicken is gold and internal temp exceeds 165°, about 45 minutes.
5. In the meantime, produce dipping sauce: In a medium dish, mix mayonnaise and hot sauce. Add more hot sauce based on desired spiciness amount.
6. Serve chicken warm with dipping sauce.

Garlic Rosemary Pork Chops:

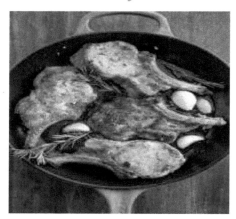

TOTAL TIME: 0 HOURS 30 MINS
YIELDS: 4
INGREDIENTS:

- 4 pieces of pork loin
- Salt (kosher)
- Black pepper freshly roasted
- 1Tbsp. of Freshly chopped rosemary
- 2 Garlic cloves, minced
- 1/2 c (1 stick) of butter melted
- 1 Tbsp. of Extra-virgin (olive oil)

DIRECTIONS:

1. Preheat the oven to 375 degrees. With salt and black pepper, season the pork chops generously.
2. Mix the honey, rosemary, and garlic together in a shallow dish. Only put back.
3. Heat the olive oil in an oven-safe skillet over (medium-high) heat and add the pork chops. Sear until golden for 4 minutes, flip and bake for a further 4 minutes. Pork chops are appropriately coated with garlic butter for 10-12 minutes.
4. Add more garlic butter to serve.

Keto Bacon Sushi

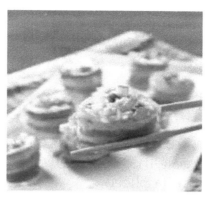

TOTAL TIME: 0 HOURS 30 MINS

YIELDS: 12

INGREDIENTS:

- 6 bacon strips, cut in half
- 2 cucumbers (Persian), cut thin
- 2 carrots (medium), cut thinly
- 1 (avocado), in slices
- 4 oz. (Creamy) cheese, cooked, soft
- Seeds of sesame (garnish)

DIRECTIONS:

1. Preheat the oven to 400 degrees. Line a baking sheet and match with a (cooling rack) with (aluminum) foil. Lay bacon half with an even surface and cook for 11 to 13 minutes unless mildly crispy but always pliable.
2. In the meantime, split the bacon's size into pieces of cucumbers, broccoli, and avocado.
3. Spread an equal surface of cream cheese from each strip until the bacon is cold enough to touch it. Divide the vegetables into the bacon equally and put them in one hand. Strictly roll up the vegetables.
4. Season with and serve the sesame seeds.

Keto Chicken Parmesan

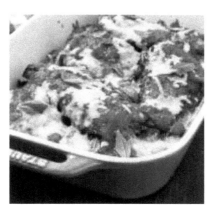

TOTAL TIME: 0 HOURS 55 MINS

YIELDS: 4

INGREDIENTS:

- 4 boneless without skin breasts of chicken
- Kosher salt
- 1c. of Almond Flour
- 3 big, beaten eggs
- 3 c. of Parmesan, freshly grated, and much more for serving
- 2 Tsp. of Powdered garlic
- 1 1/2 c. of Mozzarella Sliced
- 1 Tsp. of onion in powdered form
- 2 Tsp. of Oregano dried
- Oil for vegetables
- 3/4 c. Sugar-free, low-carb tomato sauce
- Fresh leaves of basil for topping

DIRECTIONS

1. Preheat the oven to 400 degrees. Halve the chicken breasts crosswise with a sharp knife. Season the chicken with salt and pepper on both sides.
2. Put the almond flour and eggs in 2 different shallow cups. Combine the parmesan, garlic (powder), onion (powder), and oregano in the third shallow dish. With salt and pepper, season.
3. Dip the chicken cutlets into the almond flour, then the eggs, the Parmesan mixture, and push to cover.
4. Heat 2 teaspoons of oil in a large skillet. Add chicken and roast, 2 to 3 minutes on each hand, until golden and cooked through. Function as required in batches, inserting more oil as appropriate.
5. Move the fried cutlets to a 9-inch-x-13-inch baking dish, distribute the tomato sauce uniformly over each cutlet, and finish with the mozzarella.
6. Bake for 10 to 12 minutes before the cheese melts. If needed, broil for 3 minutes until the cheese is golden.
7. Until eating, top with basil and more Parmesan.

Tuscan Butter Shrimp

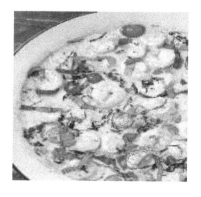

TOTAL TIME: 0 HOURS 55 MINS

YIELDS: 4

INGREDIENTS

- 2 tbsp. of olive oil extra-virgin
- 1 lb. deveined, peeled, lobster and tails cut
- salt (kosher)
- Black pepper freshly roasted
- 3 tbsp. of Butter
- 3 garlic cloves, minced
- 1 1/2 c. of halved tomatoes with cherry
- 3 c. of spinach for kids
- 1/2 c. of heavy cream
- 1/4 c. of Parmesan, finely grated
- 1/4 c. of thinly cut basil
- Lemon wedges meant for serving as an option

DIRECTIONS

1. Heat oil in a frying pan over medium heat. Season the shrimp with salt and pepper all over. Add the shrimp and sear until the underside is golden, around 2 minutes, and then turn until opaque, until the oil is shimmering but still not burning. Remove and set aside from the skillet.
2. Lower the heat to mild and add some butter. When the butter is melted, stir in the garlic and simmer for around 1 minute, until fragrant. Sprinkle with salt and substitute the cherry tomatoes. Cook until the tomatoes start to burst, then add the spinach and cook until the spinach begins to wilt.
3. Stir in the heavy cream, basil and parmesan cheese and carry the mixture to a boil. Reduce the heat to low and boil for around 3 minutes before the sauce is significantly reduced.
4. Place the shrimp back in the pan and mix to blend. Cook unless shrimp is cooked through, garnish with more basil, and squeeze lemon on top before eating.

Zoodle Alfredo with Bacon

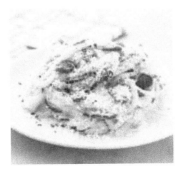

TOTAL TIME: 0 HOURS 20 MINS

YIELDS: 4

INGREDIENTS:

- 1/2 lb. of Chopped bacon
- 1 minced shallot,
- 2 garlic cloves, minced
- 1/4 c. of Black Alcohol, White Wine
- 1 1/2 c. of heavy cream
- 1/2 c. of Parmesan(cheese) grated, but mostly for garnishing
- 1 pack of zucchini (noodles) (16 oz.)
- Kosher Salt
- Black pepper freshly roast

DIRECTIONS

1. Cook the bacon until crisp, 8 minutes, in a wide saucepan over medium heat. Drain it on a tray lined with paper towels.
2. Pour all but 2 teaspoons of (bacon); then shallots are included. Cook until tender, around 2 minutes, and then add garlic and cook for about 30 seconds until it is fragrant. Add wine and cook before half the quantity is depleted.
3. Connect the heavy cream to the mixture and get it to a boil. Lower the flame and stir in the Parmesan cheese. Cook for about 2 minutes, until the sauce, has thick somewhat. Add the zucchini (noodles) and toss in the sauce until thoroughly covered. Take the heat off and stir in the fried bacon.

Keto Chicken Soup

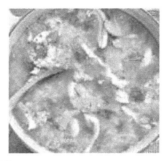

TOTAL TIME: 1 HOUR 0 MINS

YIELDS: 4 - 6

INGREDIENTS:

- 2 tbsp. Oil for vegetables
- 1 medium onion, minced
- 5 garlic cloves, crushed
- 2" Fresh ginger bit, sliced
- 1 tiny cauliflower, sliced into florets
- 3/4 Tsp. smashed flakes of red pepper
- 1 medium carrot, on a bias, peeled and thin slices
- 6 c. low-sodium broth of poultry
- 1 celery stem, thinly sliced
- 2 skinless, boneless breasts of chicken
- For garnish, finely cut parsley

DIRECTIONS

1. Heat oil in a big pot over low heat. Add the carrot, ginger, and garlic. Cook before the browning stops.
2. In the meantime, pulse cauliflower before it is split into rice-sized granules in a food processor. Return the cauliflower to the pot with the onion mixture and cook for around 8 minutes over medium-high heat until golden.
3. Bring to a boil and incorporate pepper flakes, onions, celery and chicken (broth). Add the chicken breasts and cook gently for around 15 minutes before they hit a temp of 165 ° C. Remove from the pan, leave to cool and shred until cool enough to treat. Meanwhile, proceed to cook, 3 to 5 minutes more, until the vegetables are soft.
4. Apply the (Shredded) chicken back to the broth and cut the ginger from the bath. Season with salt and pepper to taste, then garnish before serving with parsley.

Foil Pack Grilled Salmon with Lemony Asparagus

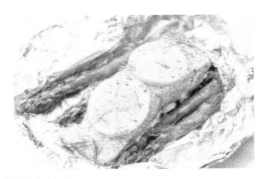

TOTAL TIME: 0 HOURS 20 MINS

YIELDS: 4

INGREDIENTS:

- 20 spears of asparagus, cut
- 4 6-oz. Skin-on fillets of salmon
- 4Tbsp. of Butter, break
- 2 lemons, cut
- Kosher salt
- Black pepper freshly roasted
- Broken dill (fresh), for season

DIRECTIONS:

1. On a hard floor lie two bits of foil. Put on the foil five spears of asparagus and finish with a salmon fillet, 1 tablespoon of butter, and two lemon slices. Cover loosely, and repeat for the rest of the ingredients and you'll have a limit of four sets.
2. High Heat Barbecue. To fry and barbecue, apply foil packets until salmon is cook through and asparagus is soft for about 10 minutes.

3. Sprinkle and mix with dill.

Garlicky Shrimp Zucchini Pasta

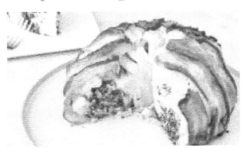

TOTAL TIME: 1 HOUR 50 MINS

YIELDS: 4

INGREDIENTS

- 1/4 c. Of olive oil extra-virgin
- 1/4 c. the Juice in Lemons
- Kosher (salt)
- 1 head (cauliflower), cut leaves and trimmed stem such that cauliflower lies flat but still intact
- 1 (10-oz.) box of frozen (spinach), thawed, stretched out and sliced with water
- 2 big, beaten eggs
- 4 green onions, cut thinly
  - 2 cloves of garlic, minced
  - 3/4 c. of cheddar Shredded
  - 4 oz. of soft and cube white cheese
  - 1/2 c. panko a panko
  - 1/4 c. of parmesan Rubbed
  - 1 lb. of bacon thinly cut

DIRECTIONS

1. Preheat the oven to 450 degrees. In a big kettle, put eight cups of water, oil, lemon juice and 2 tablespoons of salt to a boil. Add the cauliflower and get it to a simmer again. To hold it submerged, reduce it to a gentle simmer and put a plate on top of the cauliflower. Simmer for around 12 minutes before a knife is quickly inserted into the middle.
2. Transfer the cauliflower to a narrow rimmed baking sheet using 2 slotted spoons or a mesh spider. Only let it cool.
3. In the meanwhile, add lettuce (eggs, green onions, garlic, cheddar, cream cheese, panko, and parmesan cheese) and placed a 3/4-inch tip in a piping bag.
4. Place on a rimmed baking sheet with cooled cauliflower stem side up. Pipe filling of florets between stalks. Flip down the side of the cauliflower stem, and then spread bacon strips, only slightly overlapping strips, over the cauliflower, tucking strip ends into the cauliflower bottom.
5. Roast, halfway through the spinning pan, before golden all over, maybe 30 minutes.

Cajun Parmesan Salmon

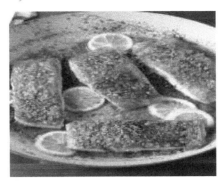

TOTAL TIME: 0 HOURS 45 MINS

YIELDS: 4

INGREDIENTS:

- 1 tbsp. Olive oil (extra-virgin)
- 4 (4-oz.) Salmon fillets (preferably wild)
- 2 Tsp. Seasoning the Cajun
- 2 Tbsp. of Butter
- 3 garlic cloves, minced
- 1/3 c. Low-sodium(chicken) or soup with vegetables
- Juice of 1 lemon
- 1 Tbsp. of honey
- 1 Tbsp. Freshly sliced parsley, with more for garnishing
- 2Tbsp. Parmesan, finely chopped
- Slices of lemon, for serving

DIRECTIONS

1. Heat oil in a frying pan over medium heat. Season the salmon with 1 tsp. of Cajun pepper and seasoning, then apply the skin-side-up to the skillet. Cook the salmon for around 6 minutes before it is intensely brown, then turn and cook for 2 more minutes. Transfer to a dish.
2. To the skillet, apply butter and garlic. Stir in the Broth, lemon juice, sugar, remaining Cajun seasoning teaspoon (parsley), and parmesan when the butter has melted. Take the combination to a boil.
3. Lower the heat to mild and return the salmon to the skillet. Simmer for 3 or 4 more minutes before the sauce is decreased, and the salmon is fried.
4. Apply slices of lemon to the pan and eat.

Beef Tenderloin:

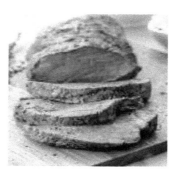

TOTAL TIME: 1 HOUR **50** MINS

YIELDS: 4

INGREDIENTS

FOR BEEF:

- 1/2 c. Olive oil (extra-virgin)
- 2 Tbsp. Vinegar (Balsamic)
- 2 Tbsp. Mustard, whole grain
- Thyme(fresh), 3 sprigs
- 3 rosemary sprigs, fresh
- 1 bay leaf
- 2 garlic cloves, crushed
- 2 tbsp. of honey
- 1 (2-lb.) tenderloin beef
- 1 Tsp. salt, Kosher
- 1 Tsp. Black pepper, roasted, fresh
- 1 Tsp. The Dried(Rosemary)
- 1 garlic clove, minced

- **SAUCE FOR YOGURT**

- 1/2 c. Yogurt (Greek)
- 1/4 c. Sour milk, sour cream
- 1 Tsp. Horseradish prepared
- 1/2 lemon extract
- Kosher salt

DIRECTIONS

1. Mix the vinegar, oil, thyme, mustard, rosemary, crushed garlic, bay leaf, and honey together in a wide container. Return the meat to the package, cover with plastic wrap, and marinate for 1 hour or up to one day in the refrigerator. Optional: Before frying, get the tenderloin to room temperature.
2. Preheat the oven to around 450C. Line an aluminum foil rimmed baking sheet and fit a wire rack inside. Strip the marinade from the tenderloin and wipe it dry with paper towels. Add salt, pepper, rosemary, and minced garlic to season all over and put on the rack.

3. Roast until baked to your taste, around 20 minutes for special occasions. Until slicing, let it rest for 5 to 10 minutes.
4. Meanwhile, render the sauce: whisk the milk, sour cream, horseradish and lemon juice together in a medium container, and season with salt.
5. Slice the tenderloin and eat it on the side with sauce.

Baked Cajun Salmon

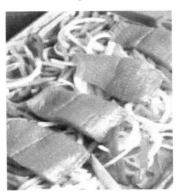

TOTAL TIME: 0 HOURS 30 MINS

YIELDS: 4

INGREDIENTS

- 1/2 large size white onion, cut thinly
- bell pepper (red), cut thinly
- 1 thinly cut orange bell pepper
- cloves of thinly sliced garlic
- Salt (kosher)
- Black Pepper, fresh, ground
- Three Tbsp. of Olive Oil (Extra-Virgin)
- 1 Tbsp. of thyme in dry form
- 1 Tbsp. of seasoning (Cajun)
- 2 Tsp. Of tweet paprika
- Tsp. of powdered garlic
- 6-oz. Filets of Salmon

DIRECTIONS:

1. Preheat the oven to 400 degrees. Stir in the onions, pepper and garlic on a   broad baking dish. Season with pepper and salt and toss with gasoline.
2. Prepare a spice mix: mix together thyme, Cajun seasoning, and paprika and garlic powder in a small cup.
3. On a baking sheet, put the salmon, top the bits with the seasoning mixture and rub them all over the salmon.
4. Bake for 20 minutes until the vegetables and salmon are soft and cooked properly.

Chapter 5: Deserts and Snacks Recipes

Keto Sugar-Free Cheesecake

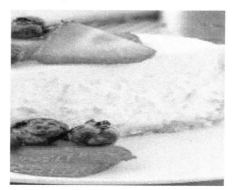

TOTAL TIME: 8 HOURS 0 MINS

YIELDS: 8 - 10

INGREDIENTS:

- 1/2 c. of almond flour
- 1/2 c. Flour of coconut
- 1/4 c. of coconut, shredded
- 1/2 c. (1 stick) of melted butter
- 3 (8-oz.) cream cheese blocks, soft to room temp
- 16 oz. of sour cream (room temperature)
- 1 Tbsp. of stevia
- 2 Tsp. a sample of pure vanilla
- 3 large size eggs, at room temperature
- Strawberries, diced, for serving

DIRECTIONS

1. Heat the oven to 300 degrees. Create the crust: Oil a spring pan of 8 or 9 inches and coat the bottom and sides with foil. Mix the rice, coconut, and butter together in a medium dish. Push the crust towards the bottom and the sides of the prepared pan somewhat upwards. When you prepare the filling, put the pan in the fridge.
2. Prepare the filling: mix together the cream cheese and sour cream in a large bowl, then whisk in the stevia and vanilla. One at a time, add the eggs, combining after each addition. Layer the filling over the crust uniformly.
3. Put the cheesecake in a deep roasting pan and set it on the oven's center rack. Pour sufficient boiling water carefully into the roasting pan to come halfway up the spring type pan's sides. Bake for 1 hour to 1 hour 20 minutes, until the middle jiggles just slightly. Switch off the oven, but allow the cake to cool steadily for an hour in the oven with the door partially closed.

4. Remove the pan from the boiling water, remove the foil, and then let it cool for at least five hours or overnight in the refrigerator. Slice with the strawberries and garnish.

Keto Chocolate Chip Cookies

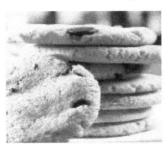

TOTAL TIME: 0 HOURS 30 MINS

YIELDS: 18

INGREDIENTS:

- 2 large size eggs
- 1/2 c (1 stick) of butter that has melted
- 2 Tbsp. of heavy milk to heavy cream
- 2 Tsp .pure extract of vanilla
- 2 3/4 c. of almond flour
- 1/4 Tsp. salt, kosher
- 1/4 c. Sugar granulated keto-friendly (such as swerve)
- 3/4 c. Chips of dark chocolate (such as lily's)
- cooking mist

DIRECTIONS

1. Preheat 350° in the oven. Mix the egg with the sugar, vanilla and heavy cream in a big dish. Add the almond flour, salt and swerve to the mixture.
2. Fold in the cookie batter with the chocolate chips. Shape the mixture into 1" balls and arrange 3" apart on baking sheets lined with parchment. Flatten the balls with cooking spray on the bottom of a glass that has been oiled.
3. Bake for around 17 to 19 minutes until the cookies are softly golden.

Keto Chocolate Mug Cake

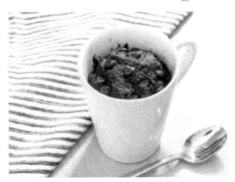

TOTAL TIME: 0 HOURS 5 MINS

YIELDS: 1

INGREDIENTS:

- 2 Tbsp. of Butter
- 1/4 c. of almond flour
- 2 Tbsp. of powdered cocoa
- 1 large size egg, beaten
- 2 Tbsp. of chocolate chips that are keto-friendly, (such as Lily's)
- 2 Tbsp. of Swerve, Granulated
- 1/2 Tsp. of baking powder
- A pinch of Kosher salt
- For serving, whipped cream (1/4 c.)

DIRECTIONS

1. Put the butter in a microwave-safe mug and heat for 30 seconds before it is melted. Except for whipped cream, add the remaining ingredients and stir until thoroughly mixed. Cook until the cake is set, but always fudgy, for 45 seconds to 1 minute.
2. Serve with whipped cream.

Keto Ice Cream

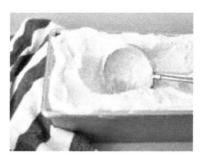

TOTAL TIME: 8 HOURS 15 MINS

YIELDS: 8

INGREDIENT:

- 2 cans of coconut milk (15-oz.)
- 2 c. of heavy cream
- 1/4 c. Swerve the Sweetener of the Confectioner
- 1 Tsp. of pure vanilla
- A pinch of Kosher salt

DIRECTIONS

1. In the refrigerator, chill the coconut milk for at least 3 hours, preferably overnight.
2. To make whipped coconut: pour coconut cream into a big bowl, keep liquid in the bowl and beat the coconut cream until very smooth using a hand mixer. Only put back.
3. Make the whipped cream: Using a hand mixer in a separate big bowl (or a stand mixer in a bowl), beat heavy cream until soft peaks shape. Beat in the vanilla and sweetener.
4. Fold the whipped (coconut) into the whipped cream, and then add the mixture to the loaf plate.
5. Freeze for about 5 hours until it is firm.

Keto Hot Chocolate

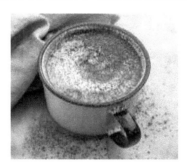

TOTAL TIME: 0 HOURS 10 MINS

YIELDS: 1 CUP

INGREDIENTS:

- 2 Tbsp. Powder of unsweetened chocolate, and more for garnishing
- 2 1/2 Tsp. of sugar that is keto-friendly, such as Swerve
- 1 1/4 c. Aquatic Water
- 1/4 c. Heavy milk to heavy cream
- 1/4 Tsp. of pure vanilla
- Whipped(milk),for serving

DIRECTIONS:

1. Whisk together the swerve, chocolate, and about 2 teaspoons of water in a shallow pan over medium heat until smoother and dissolve. Increases heat to low, add the remaining cream and water and whisk until heated regularly.
2. Attach the vanilla, and spill it into a cup. Represent with (whipped) cream and chocolate powder dusting.

Keto Peanut Butter Cookies

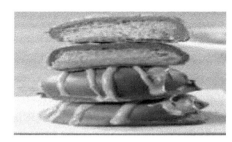

TOTAL TIME: 1 HOUR 30 MINS

YIELDS: 22

INGREDIENTS

- 1 1/2c. of smooth peanut butter, unsweetened, melted (plus more for drizzling)
- 1 c. Flour of coconut
- 1/4 c. Keto-friendly brown sugar packets, such as Swerve
- 1 Tsp. of pure vanilla
- Pinch of Kosher salt
- 2 c. of melted keto-friendly dark chocolate chips, including Lily's,
- 1 Tbsp. of Cream (Coconut)
-

DIRECTIONS

1. Combine the sugar, coconut flour, peanut butter, salt, and vanilla in a medium dish. Until smooth, stir.
2. Line the parchment paper with a baking sheet. Shape the mixture into circles using a small cookie scoop, then push down gently to flatten slightly and position it on the baking sheet. Freeze until strong, roughly 1 hour.
3. Whisk the melting chocolate and coconut oil together in a medium dish.
4. Dip peanut butter rounds in chocolate using a fork until fully covered and then return to the baking sheet. Drizzle with much more peanut butter, and freeze for around 10 minutes before the chocolate is set.
5. Only serve it cold. In the fridge, put some leftovers.

Chocolate Keto Cookies

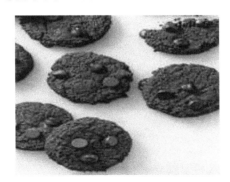

TOTAL TIME: 0 HOURS 25 MINS

YIELDS: 11

INGREDIENTS

- 2 1/2 Tbsp. of butter
- 3 Tbsp. of chocolate chips with keto, split
- 1large size egg
- 1 Tsp. of pure vanilla
- 2/3 of c. Almond Flour Blanched
- 1/3 c. of swerve Confectioners
- 3 1/2 Tbsp. Unsweetened dark chocolate powder
- 1/2 Tsp. Powder used for baking
- Pinch of Kosher salt

DIRECTIONS

1. Preheat the oven to 325 degrees. Add butter and half of the (chocolate chips) into a medium-sized dish. Microwave for 15 to 30 seconds, only enough time to melt the chocolate and butter mildly. Until a chocolate sauce emerges, mix the two together.
2. Attach and whisk the egg in a tiny dish before the yolk mixes with the whites. When it's finished, add the chocolate syrup to the bowl with the egg and vanilla extract. Again, blend.
3. To finish the cookies, add the majority of the dry ingredients, save some of the chocolate chips. Mix until it shapes a mass of chocolate cookie dough.
4. To make 11 equal-sized cookies, use a cookie spoon (or a tablespoon). Attach the cookie to a baking parchment paper and top the remainder of the chocolate chips with each cookie. In either a spoon or a spatula, flatten each cookie.
5. For 8 to 10 minutes, roast. When they come out of the oven, they should be very soft, but don't worry, this is natural!
6. Let the cookies on the baking sheet cool off. They can set up and firm up while they cool up.
7. When the leftovers are cooled, enjoy them and store them in an airtight jar in the refrigerator.

Walnut Snowball Cookies:

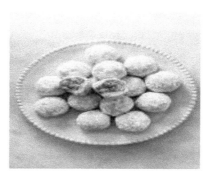

TOTAL TIME: 1 HOUR 5 MINS

YIELDS: 15

INGREDIENTS

- 1/2 c. (1 stick) of butter that has melted
- 1 large size egg
- 50 drops of stevia liquid (about 1/4 tsp.)
- 1/2 tsp. of pure vanilla
- 1 c. With walnuts
- 1/2 c. Flour of coconut, plus 1 or 2 tbsp. For rolling, more
- 1/2 c. of swerve Confectioners

DIRECTIONS

1. Preheat the oven to 300 ° and use parchment paper to cover a baking sheet. In a large bowl, mix the melted butter, egg, vanilla extract, stevia and set aside.
2. In a food processor, add the walnuts and pulse until ground. In a medium bowl, pour the walnut flour and add the coconut flour and 1/4 cup Swerve and press until mixed.
3. Add the dry mixture to the wet in two sections and whisk to blend. The dough should be soft but strong enough at this stage to shape hand-made balls without sticking to your hands. If the quality is not right, add 1 to 2 tablespoons of extra (coconut) flour and mix.
4. Create 15 balls of the same size and place them on a lined baking sheet. In the microwave, they would not disperse.
5. For 30 minutes, roast.
6. Enable 5 minutes to settle, and then in the remaining 1/4 cup Swerve, roll the (still warm) spheres.
7. Put them back on the parchment paper and give another 20 to 30 minutes to cool fully before feeding.

Keto Tortilla Chips

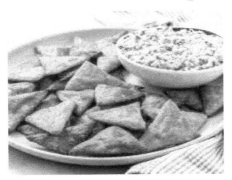

TOTAL TIME: 0 HOURS 35 MINS

YIELDS: 4 - 6

INGREDIENTS

- 2 c. of Mozzarella cheese, Sliced
- 1 c. of almond flour
- 1 Tsp. salt, Kosher
- 1 Tsp. of garlic powder
- 1/2 Tsp. Powdered chili
- Black pepper freshly ground

DIRECTIONS

1. Preheat the oven to 350 degrees. Top the parchment paper with two wide baking sheets.
2. Melt the mozzarella in a secure microwave bowl for around 1 minute and 30 seconds. Add the almond flour, cinnamon, chili powder, garlic powder, black pepper and a few pieces. Use both hands to moisten the dough a couple of times before it forms a smooth shape.
3. Place the dough between two parchment paper sheets and stretch it out into a 1/8' wide rectangle. Break the dough into triangles using a knife or a pizza cutter.
4. Spread the chips on lined baking sheets and bake for 12 to 14 minutes until the sides are golden and begin to crisp.

Keto Burger Fat Bombs

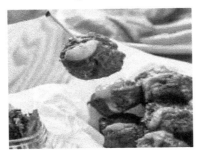

TOTAL TIME: 0 HOURS 30 MINS

YIELDS: 20

INGREDIENTS:

- Cooking mist
- 1 lb. of meat, ground
- 1/2 tsp. powder in garlic form
- salt (kosher)
- Black pepper freshly ground
- 2 tbsp. Cold butter, 20 bits of sliced butter
- 2 oz. Split into 20 bits of cheddar,
- Lettuce berries meant for serving
- For serving, finely sliced tomatoes
- Mustard, to serve

DIRECTIONS

1. Preheat the oven to 375 °C and oil the cooking spray with a mini muffin tin. Season the beef with salt, garlic powder and pepper in a medium dish.
2. Place 1 teaspoon of beef equally, covering the bottom entirely, into the bottom of each muffin tin cup. Place a slice of butter on top and press 1 teaspoon of beef over the butter to cover full.
3. In each cup, place a slice of cheddar on top of the meat and force the remaining beef over the cheese to cover it fully.
4. Bake for about 15 minutes before the meat is ready. Let yourself cool somewhat.
5. Using a metal offset spatula carefully to release each burger out of the tin. Serve with onions, salad leaves, and mustard.

Jalapeño Popper Egg Cups

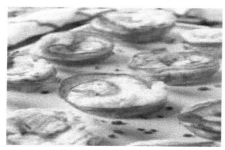

TOTAL TIME: 0 HOURS 45 MINS

YIELDS: 12

INGREDIENTS:

- 12 strips of bacon
- 10 eggs (large)
- 1/4 c. of sour milk,
- 1/2 c. Cheddar Shredded
- 1/2 c. Mozzarella Sliced
- 2(jalapeños), 1 sliced thinly and 1 finely chopped
- 1 Tsp. Powdered of garlic
- salt(kosher)

- Black pepper freshly ground
- Cooking spray, nonstick

DIRECTIONS

1. Preheat the oven to 375 degrees. Over medium heat, (cook bacon) in a broad skillet until well browned but always pliable. Put aside to drain on a paper towel-lined pan.
2. Whisk the eggs, sour cream, cheese, minced jalapeño and garlic in powder form together in a big bowl. With salt and pepper, season.
3. Oil a muffin tin with the aid of nonstick cooking oil. Line each well with one bacon strip, then pour each muffin cup with egg mixture until around two-thirds of the way through to the end. Cover each muffin with a slice of jalapeño.
4. Bake for 20 minutes until the eggs do not look moist anymore. Before withdrawing them from the muffin pan, cool slightly.

Keto Frosty

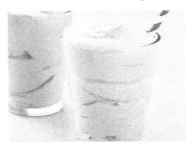

TOTAL TIME: 0 HOURS 45 MINS

YIELDS: 4

INGREDIENTS

- 1 1/2 c. Heavy cream whipping
- 2 Tbsp. Unsweetened powder of cocoa
- 3 Tbsp. Sweetener for (keto-friendly) powdered sugar, such as a Swerve
- 1 Tsp. of pure vanilla
- Pinch of Kosher salt

DIRECTIONS

1. Combine the milk, sugar, sweetener, vanilla, and salt in a wide pot. Beat the mixture until rigid peaks shape, and use a hand blender or (the whisk attachment of a stand mixer). Mix the scoops into a Ziploc container and ice for 30 to 35 minutes before they're frozen.
2. Break the tip off an edge of the Ziploc container and pour it into dishes to eat.

Bacon Guac Bombs

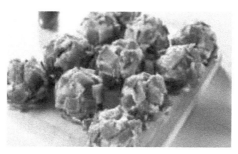

TOTAL TIME: 0 HOURS 45 MINS
YIELDS: 15
INGREDIENTS:

2 bacon strips, fried and crumbled

For guacamole

- 2 pitted, sliced, and mashed avocados
- 6 oz. of Cream cheese, cooked, softened
- 1 lime juice
- 1 clove of garlic, minced
- 1/4 of red onion, minced
- 1 small jalapeno (seeded if less fire is preferred), chopped
- 2 Tbsp. Cilantro, freshly sliced
- 1/2 Tsp. of cumin seeds
- 1/2 Tsp. Powdered of chili
- salt(kosher)
- Black pepper freshly ground

DIRECTIONS

1. Combine all the guacamole products in a big bowl. Stir unless mostly smooth, and add salt and pepper (some pieces are OK). Put in the freezer for 30 minutes to firm up rapidly.

2. On a wide tray, put crumbled bacon. Scoop the guacamole mix and put in the bacon, utilizing a little cookie scoop. Roll in the bacon to coat. Repeat before you've used both the bacon and guacamole. Store in refrigerator.

Avocado Chips

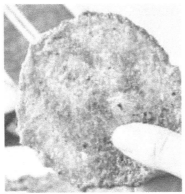

TOTAL TIME: 0 HOURS 40 MINS
YIELDS: 15
INGREDIENTS

- 1 large ripe avocado
- 3/4 c. Freshly grated parmesan
- 1 tsp. Lemon juice
- 1/2 tsp. Garlic powder
- 1/2 tsp. Italian seasoning
- Kosher salt
- Freshly ground black pepper

DIRECTIONS

1. Preheat oven to 325° and line two baking sheets with parchment paper. In a medium bowl, mash avocado with a fork until smooth. Stir in parmesan, lemon juice, garlic powder, and Italian seasoning. Season with salt and pepper.
2. Place heaping teaspoon-size scoops of mixture on baking sheet, leaving about 3" apart between each scoop. Flatten each scoop to 3" wide across with the back of a spoon or measuring cup. Bake until crisp and golden, about 30 minutes, then let cool completely. Serve at room temperature.

Rosemary Keto Crackers

TOTAL TIME: 1 HOUR 0 MINS
YIELDS: 140
INGREDIENTS

- 2 1/2 c. almond flour
- 1/2 c. coconut flour
- 1 tsp. ground flaxseed meal
- 1/2 tsp. dried rosemary, chopped
- 1/2 tsp. onion powder
- 1/4 tsp. kosher salt
- 3 large eggs
- 1 tbsp. extra-virgin olive oil

DIRECTIONS

1. Preheat oven to 325° and line a baking sheet with parchment paper. In a large bowl, whisk together flours, flaxmeal, rosemary, onion powder, and salt. Add eggs and oil and mix to combine. Continue mixing until dough forms a large ball, about 1 minute.
2. Sandwich dough between 2 pieces of parchment and roll to ¼" thick. Cut into squares and transfer to prepared baking sheet.
3. Bake until golden, 12 to 15 minutes. Let cool before storing in a resalable container.

Conclusion

A ketogenic diet could be an alternative for certain people who have experienced trouble losing weight with other approaches. The exact ratio of fat, carbohydrate, and protein that is required to attain health benefits can differ among individuals due to their genetic makeup and body structure. Therefore, if one decides to start a ketogenic diet, it is advised to meet with one's physician and a dietitian to closely track any metabolic adjustments since beginning the treatment and to develop a meal schedule that is specific to one's current health problems and to avoid food shortages or other health risks. A dietitian can also have advice on reintroducing carbs after weight reduction is accomplished.

The 15-Day Keto Fasting Cookbook

A Sophisticated Mix of Low-Carb Recipes to Activate Ketosis and Autophagy for Life-Long Intermittent Fasting

By

Gianna Carter

Contents

Introduction

Given the multiple kinds of diets you have probably read about in your life, you are likely to have a few fresh ones. Perhaps one amongst them may be the Ketogenic Diet, commonly known as the Keto Diet, which is a low-carbohydrate, high-fat regimen.

The idea behind the high-fat, low-carbohydrate ratio is that instead of carbs, the body would depend on fats for nutrition, and hence the body would become leaner as a consequence of getting less fat contained throughout the body.

Ideally, the Keto Diet would encourage the body to achieve ketosis or a metabolic condition where the carbs are ketones, which are fats that are burned for energy rather than glucose. Many who embrace the Keto Diet often eat only the correct amount of protein on a regular basis that the body requires. The Keto Diet does not rely on measuring calories, compared to any of the other diets that occur. Instead, the emphasis is on the food's fat, proteins and carbohydrates make-up, as well as the weight of the servings.

But what contributed to the Keto Diet being created?

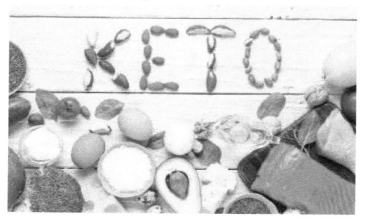

In hopes of discovering a cure for seizures, a Mayo Clinic physician by the name of Russell Wilder invented the Ketogenic Diet back in 1924. Since going on this diet, many people who have epilepsy and other disorders have reported a substantial reduction in their symptoms. This procedure goes back to Ancient Greece when physicians would change the diets of their patients and even make them rapidly push their bodies into hunger mode.

The Ketogenic Diet is a much better way for the body to reach the fasting mode without completely depriving the body of food. However, to this day, no one understands precisely why the Ketogenic Diet is so effective in treating those who have epilepsy, autism, and other identified diseases.

The high-fat, low-carbohydrate combination might be a normal meal for those on the Ketogenic Diet, which would include a balanced portion of some fruit or a protein-rich vegetable, protein such as chicken and a high-fat portion that may be butter. The high-fat portion of this diet typically comes from the food-making ingredients; this may involve heavy cream, butter, or buttermilk, and creamy dressings such as ranch could also be mixed.

Unfortunately, with its potential for instantaneous results, this natural approach to healing had to give way to the new advancement of medicinal research.

Happily, again and perhaps for really good purposes, the ketogenic diet has made its way back into the spotlight!

You see, the cornerstone of the diet is to effectively stimulate the fat-burning processes of your own body to feel what the body wants for energy during the day. This implies that all the fat you consume and the accumulated fat in your body have both been fuel reserves that can be taped over by your body! No wonder that except among some persistent, hard to lose fat regions, this plan also helps you with weight reduction. It may be one of the explanations why you selected this eBook and looked into the ketogenic process, or you might have learned stories from your social group on how the keto diet really normalizes blood glucose levels and optimizes the cholesterol measurements and you are fascinated. Only by adopting this plan alone, how about the news of type 2 diabetes getting cured as well as stories of some diseases being prevented or tumors shrinking thanks to the beneficial impact of the keto diet? Even as a result of the diet, we do overlook the risk of heart disease!

All the above-mentioned advantages derive primarily from a single major mechanism in the ketogenic diet. The name of the game is ketosis.

In this very book, all information about the keto diet and intermittent fasting is provided and lets you know how it's helpful for quick and healthy weight loss.

Chapter 1- Ketogenic Diet and Ketosis

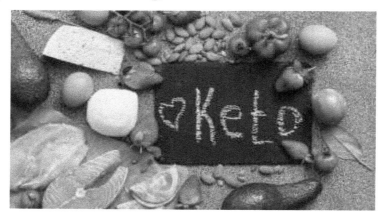

You may be on a ketogenic diet or are contemplating it.

If you desire to kickstart with ketosis, then your ticket is for intermittent fasting.

Truth be known, it can be daunting to follow a ketogenic diet, mainly because there are too many things that you cannot consume. But be assured the truth-ketosis is spiritual.

Fortunately, whether you don't want to eat a ketogenic diet, you will easily get a route to ketosis.

When the body burns up ketones and fat for food instead of glucose, ketosis happens.

In two cases, that happens:

1. there is no food coming (fasting) or
2. little or no carbohydrates come through (ketogenic dieting).

It regularly makes ketones in the process when your system is in the fat-burning phase; hence, you are in ketosis.

For the body to be in the process of ketosis is perfectly natural, and it was definitely a popular occurrence for humans across history that had intermittent accessibility to food and fasting times in between. For those following a Western diet, though, the physiological condition of ketosis is very unusual since we are all feeding. You basically get negligible ketones in your blood while you're consuming something else than a ketogenic diet. But it's very rare for our generation of people to be in a condition of ketosis unless you seek one out purposefully.

Post 8 hours of fasting, as you wake up, ketone levels are only starting to raise. Ketone output will speed up to provide more of the energy you need if you prolong your fast until noon, and your body will finally be in the renowned fat-burning condition of ketosis. If you want to manage to burn body fat at a high pace by keeping to your fast for 16 hours or a day or a few days, and not by consuming anything ketogenic, you need to live in ketosis!

A lot of focus is given to reaching ketosis through ketogenic diets, but if you consume keto foods, where do you suppose any of the ketones come from? And not the fat on the thighs and hips. Fasting for ketosis means that only the body fat comes from the ketones that feed the brain, thereby getting rid of it.

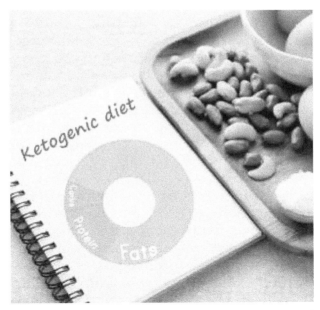

Ketosis is a condition in which the body creates compounds that are formed by the liver, labeled ketones. Crafted to supply organs and cells with nutrition, it may substitute sugar as an additional source of food. We get much of our energy from glucose in our conventional diet, rich in carbs which are processed from the carbohydrates that we consume throughout meals. Glucose is a fast energy supply, where insulin is needed as a kind of intermediary that tells the cells to open up and enables the flow of glucose so that it can be used as a mitochondrial fuel, better known as the fuel factories in our cells. The further sugars we eat, the more glucose is found in our blood, which suggests that the pancreas has to generate more insulin to promote the extraction of energy from usable blood sugar. In an organism where the metabolism is still natural, the cells readily embrace the insulin released by the pancreas, which then contributes to the effective use of blood glucose as energy. The concern is that our cells will actually become desensitized to insulin, contributing to a condition in which the pancreas is required to inject more and more insulin into the bloodstream only to clear the blood sugar levels and normalize them.

Insulin de-sensitivity or insulin tolerance is primarily induced by the constant enhanced presence of blood glucose and is typically caused by the intake of foods high in carbon. Picture of the cells of the body like a security guard at a bar, where you need to pay a charge to enter the club. Here, you play a glucose function, and the cost paid to join the club is insulin. If the club intensity is in accordance with the standard, the security officer doesn't really notice something odd and does not increase the admission fee needed. However, if you wake up clamoring to be allowed in just about every night, the bouncer understands the dire need and jacks up the insulin charge periodically in order to let glucose in. Gradually, at such a stage that the source of insulin, which in this situation is the pancreas, no longer generates any, the admission fee grows greater and greater. This is when the situation is diagnosed with type 2 diabetes, and the normal solution will include drugs or insulin injections for a lifetime. In the existence of glucose in the body system lies the crux of the matter here. Our blood sugar levels are raised every time we take in a carb-rich meal, which is not complicated in this day and age of fast food and sugary snacks, and insulin is enabled for the conversion into energy as well as the storage of the wasted waste into fat cells. This is where the normal furor begins, with condemnations pouring in as the cause of numerous ailments and dreaded weight gain with both glucose and insulin. It wouldn't be wrong if it claimed that insulin and glucose, as certain books have made them out to be, are most certainly not the source of all bad. To refer to our present diet as the leading cause of metabolic disorders and obesity plaguing the greater part of the developing world will be much more specific.

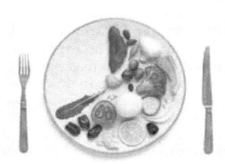

Link the ketogenic diet, which is where the shift toward the positive will be seen.

The keto diet, with a focus on being intentionally low carb, is a fat-based diet. This strategy is intended to decrease our consumption of sugar and starchy foods that are too easily affordable. Just a pleasant fact: in the old days, sugar was actually used as a preservative, and it's no accident that a number of the packaged goods we have now involve massive quantities of sugar so that it makes for longer shelf life. The hedonic appetite reaction in the brain has often been found to cause foods rich in sugar, ultimately allowing you to feed for the sake of gratification rather than actual hunger. Studies also found that sugar therapies are linked to the regions of the brain that are often responsible for opioid use and gambling. You know now that it appears like you can't resist tossing those caramelized sweets into the mouth.

So, we cut back on sugars, and this is where the fat comes in to offset the calories required to help the body. You will be looking at taking seventy-five percent of the daily calorie as fats on the regular ketogenic diet, approximately twenty percent as protein and the remaining five percent in the form of carbohydrates. We are doing it because, as we know, we want our key source of fuel to be fat. We will cause the body to induce ketosis only with the mixture of cutting down carbohydrates and growing our fat intake. We either do so with a diet that makes long-term, safe use, or we actually starve through ketosis. Yeah, sure, you heard it correctly; ketosis is the normal mechanism of the body that creates a shield against the lean periods where there is a lack   of   food.

Chapter 2- Intermittent fasting and the ketogenic diet

In recent years, this has also been bandied about a lot, with some seeking to shed a misleading light on the keto diet by associating it with thirst.

To make it simpler, when our bodies feel that we do not have adequate glucose in the bloodstream, the ketosis mechanism is initiated. In order to ensure the continuous availability of nutrition for our cells and tissues, it then switches to our fat reserves to transform them into ketones via the liver. It does not mean that you are necessarily killing yourself on the keto diet! Any time someone says that, he got a little worked up.

How will a person who eats 1,800 to 2,000 calories on a regular basis, which is what you're going to get on the meal plan, starve effectively?

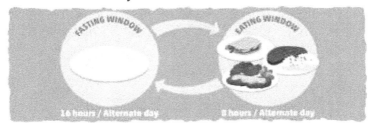

To be fair, during the hunter-gatherer days of our human past, ketosis comes in very handy. This was a time where agriculture wasn't that common, and what you searched or found relied on the food you consumed. This produced a scenario where there could be no calories for days at a time, so our bodies sent insulin to ferry it through our organs as glucose made its way through the environment, as well as hoarding the leftover glucose into fat cells for potential usage.

The body then reached the condition of ketosis by using the accumulated fats to provide nutrition during the lean periods when there was really little food to be found.

Our hunger hormones, like ghrelin, decrease their development during this stage, and the hormones that regulate satiety, like leptin, see their levels increased. All this is how our bodies want to make the most of it to make it easier for us to feel as comfortable as possible if nutritional supplies are scarce.

Today, quick forward to modern days, where food is practically only one or two streets away, or maybe just a car ride away, and we're not going to experience food scarcity like our predecessors in the Paleolithic. However, our bodies also retain the processes and pathways that have enabled them to function. That is the main explanation why we reduce carbohydrates and raise our regular fat consumption on the keto diet.

The condition of ketosis is triggered when we do so, and we get to reap all the biochemical advantages that the diet confers.

The fat we consume often goes into replenishing the body's fat reserves, which is why it won't be wrong to claim again when on the ketogenic diet, one should not starve!

How the Intermitting Fasting Works

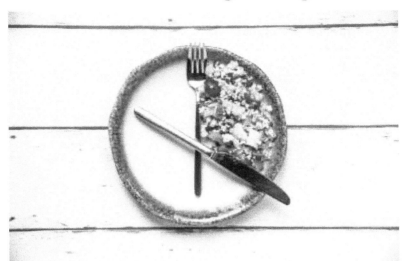

From the context of weight reduction, intermittent fasting operates by finding it more challenging to overeat during the day. A basic guideline such as "skip breakfast" or "eat only between 5 pm and 8 pm" will help keep you from reaching for sweets or consuming calorie-dense drinks that lead to weight gain during the day.

You'll also find it impossible to overeat, even though you work up a ferocious appetite when fasting. In fact, intermittent fasting appears to decrease the intake of daily energy and encourage fat loss.

This ensures that as long as you adhere to a shorter feeding time or a fixed number of meals, you can be willing to consume as much as you like and meet your objectives.

Your body may need to adapt itself to this new eating pattern when you first attempt intermittent fasting. Hunger pangs and strong cravings may strike you hard at first, but they will soon recede when your cells feast on accumulated fat and ketones.

Insulin removal, ketone synthesis and autophagy are the main pathways behind your ability to quickly lose weight and boost your health in the process. Our insulin levels drop incrementally as we accumulate time in a fasting condition. This facilitates the liberation of fat from our fat cells and activates the mechanism known as ketogenesis that generates ketones.

You'll reach a deeper state of ketosis as you continue your easy, become more successful at burning fat, and speed up the self-cleaning mechanism known as autophagy.

Benefits of Intermitting Fasting

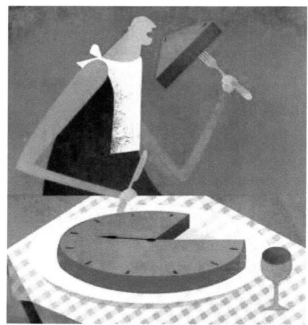

1. Enhanced regulation of blood sugar and resistance to insulin

This will also help boost blood sugar levels and improve one's cells' insulin response by allowing the body an occasional break from calorie intake. One research study showed that for six meals a day, intermittent fasting could also be a healthier option than having the same calorie deficit.

The two dietary strategies can function synergistically to boost blood sugar regulation when paired with the keto diet, which has also been shown to assist with insulin tolerance and type 2 diabetes. More study on the results of using them in tandem, however, is needed.

2. Psychic Clarity

Your brain will essentially operate on ketones, which are extracted through fat dissolution in the liver until the body is keto-adapted.

Fat is thought to be one of the body's most energy-efficient resources to work on, and your mind is a major energy user.

When you do not regularly refill on grains and fruits, most high-carb supporters fight for the malnutrition your body endures. They expect you to take a granola bar and an apple around you everywhere you go, but the advantage of Keto is that you don't.

And if the body is full of glycogen (which is more definitely if you are in ketosis), the excess of fat from the meals you consume and shop you have will depend on it. That ensures that your brain powerhouse will operate at maximum capacity all the time. Less emotional fogginess and more attention.

You can begin to lose fat automatically when you get used to dieting. In other terms, feed only when you are starving. Don't arrange the fasting; let it arise spontaneously.

3. Fitness

People still claim that if you don't use the benefit of pre-and post-exercise meals while you work out, you're going to lose muscle.

This is not inherently real, and when you're adapted to ketosis, it is much less so.

In the long run, fasting while practicing can contribute to a variety of advantages, including:

1. **Greater mutation adaptations** - Studies indicate that when you work out in a fasting condition, your training efficiency will improve in the long run.
2. **Enhanced muscle synthesis-** Experiments indicate that when you exercise in a fasting condition and use sufficient nutrient consumption, muscle gains are improved.
3. **Increased reaction to post-workout meals-**Studies suggests that the accelerated ingestion of nutrients after a short exercise will contribute to better outcomes.

Mechanism Behind the Benefits

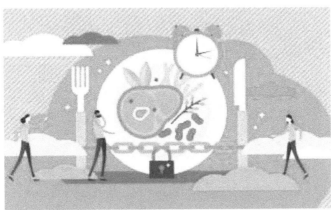

Intermittent fasting is so effective that it can be used to reduce calories, trigger ketosis, and enable the mechanisms of autophagy induced by protein restriction and hunger.

This is what happens to our cells as we consume three or more meals a day, which meets our normal calorie requirements fully. Your cells will also be backed up with non-essential proteins and poisonous chemicals, sometimes after consuming the healthiest diets, but what can you do?

You soon, not from cooking, but from being consumed by other commitments, to ensure you clean your real bedroom. You need to fast with food to ensure sure the cells will clean themselves.

Not only can this fasting phase trigger this cleanup for your cells, but it will increase the output of your ketones and facilitate fat burning as well. Simply stated, by incorporating intermittent fasting into the keto diet, coupled with the consequences of autophagy, you can enjoy the advantages of Keto more easily.

In addition, you will raise ketone amounts, lose more fat, and improve autophagy more than you can with intermittent fasting alone if you begin to implement intermittent fasting and exercise together.

Overall, the evidence for intermittent fasting shows that it will be a perfect complement to the keto lifestyle for certain persons, whether you include activity or not. Before you start, though, it is important to be acquainted with the unpleasant signs that can occur.

Chapter 3- How autophagy and ketosis are synergic?

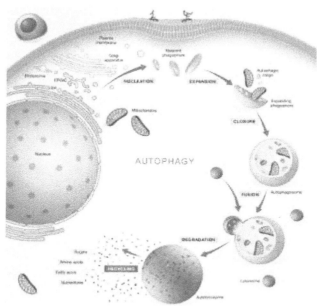

In order to reconstruct healthy, healthier cells, autophagy is the body's method of wiping out dead cells.

Auto" implies self, and "phagy" implies eating." So, 'self-eating' is the literal sense of autophagy.

That is often referred to as "self-devouring." Although it might seem like something you would wish to occur to your body, your ultimate wellbeing is actually advantageous.

It is since autophagy is an evolved method of self-preservation by which the organism can extract and regenerate sections of dysfunctional cells for cellular repair and hygiene.

The aim of autophagy is to eliminate debris and return to optimum smooth operation through self-regulation.

Around the same moment, it's recycling and washing, almost like touching the body on a reset button. Plus, as a reaction to different stressors and contaminants accumulated in our bodies, it encourages resilience and adaptation.

Note that autophagy simply means "self-eating." Therefore, it makes sense that it is understood that intermittent fasting and ketogenic diets induce autophagy.

The most successful method to cause autophagy is by fasting.

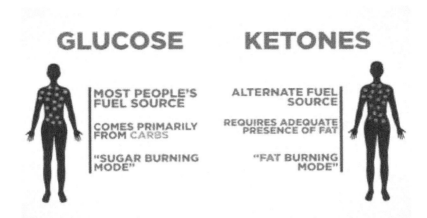

Ketosis, a high-fat and low-carb diet, offers the same advantages to eating without fasting, such as a shortcut that causes the same advantageous biochemical adjustments. It allows the body a break to concentrate on its own wellbeing and repair by not stressing the body with an external load.

You receive about 75 percent of the recommended daily calories from fat in the keto diet and 5 to 10 percent of your calories from carbohydrates.

This alteration in calorie sources allows the biochemical processes in the body to change. Instead of the glucose that is extracted from carbohydrates, it would start using fat for food.

In reaction to this ban, the body will begin to start creating ketone bodies that have several protective effects. Khorana says studies show that ketosis, which has neuroprotective functions, may also cause starvation-induced autophagy.

In all diets, low glucose levels exist and are related to low insulin and high levels of glucagon. And the degree of glucagon is the one that initiates autophagy.

It brings the constructive stress that wakes up the survival repair mode when the body is low on sugar by fasting or ketosis.

Exercise is one non-diet region that can also play a part in causing autophagy. Physical activity can, according to one animal research, cause autophagy in organs that are part of the processes of metabolic control.

Chapter 4- Keto Diet and weight loss

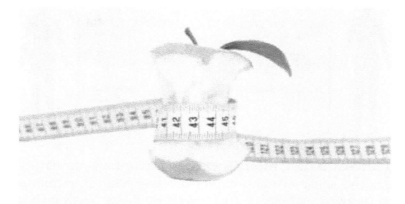

When we start on a ketogenic diet, one of the first items we still lose is most certainly water weight. As adipose fats, the body stores glucose, although there is a limited supply of glucose that is processed as glycogen, composed mainly of water. Glycogen is intended to provide rapid bursting capacity, the kind we use when we run or raise weights. The body switches to glycogen as the first source of energy supply as we cut carbohydrates, which is why water weight is lost in the initial phases. This initial blast of weight reduction may be a morale booster for everyone, and for people who conform to the keto diet, it is a positive signpost for what is to come. Water weight is readily lost and gained, as a side note. This suggests that even those who first see certain outcomes in the keto diet and then wish to get off the track for some reason, as carbohydrates become the daily calorie mainstay, the odds are their weight would swell back up.

For the rest that conforms to the ketogenic diet, what comes next will be the fat burning process of the body that is responsible for the impressive effects of weight loss shown by many. The underlying principle is also the same in that adipose fats are still activated by the organs and cells of the body as energy sources, contributing to a normal state of depletion of fat and thus accompanying reducing weight.

The burning of fat is not the sole explanation that the keto diet demonstrates weight reduction.

Hunger reduction and improvement of pleasure during meals are also explanations that people are better able to lose weight whilst on a diet. One of the long-standing ideals of weight management has always been the adage of drinking less and doing more. The entire premise is to establish a calorie shortage in such a way that the body is forced to depend on its stored energy reserves to make up for the requisite expenditure. That seems quick and straightforward on paper, but it may be as challenging as scaling Mount Everest for someone who has been through scenarios where you have had to deliberately curtail your food on a hungry stomach!

Through the ketogenic diet, thanks to the modification of the hormones that regulate sensations of appetite and fullness, you realize that you will have normal hunger suppression. In addition, the food we usually eat while on a diet often assists with weight reduction. It is understood that fats and protein are more relaxing and rewarding than sugary carbs. We do two items almost concurrently as we turn to a high-fat diet when cutting back on the carbohydrates. Only because we feel like it, not because we are very hungry, easing back on carbohydrates, particularly the sugar stuff, reduces the urge to consume. Charging high the consumption of fat often causes the satiety impact even easier and helps you to feel complete. This is part of so many keto dieters claim that without having the smallest pinch of hunger, they will go for two and a half or even two meals a day.

We account for a regular caloric consumption that varies from 1,800 to 2,000 calories on our keto meal schedule, but we do not even use calorie limits to minimize weight. The truth is that those tiny and harmless-looking snacks that fill the period between dinners will not appear much in your life when you feel fullness and enjoyment from your meals! Think about it: the usual go-to sweets, donuts, candy, and cookies, are left out purely, so you are less inclined to give in to hedonistic appetite induced mainly by the same sugar treats in reducing extra calories which would have otherwise been converted to adipose fat tissue, that goes a very long way.

To sum up, without the usual calorie limit in most weight reduction diets, the ketogenic diet provides for meals. It also offers a supporting hand in the production of symptoms of hunger suppression such that you do not have to struggle with those treacherous hunger pangs! The lack of carb munchies is also present, which may theoretically disrupt any diet. With as minimal disturbance to our everyday life as possible, this helps one to experience normal weight loss. There is no need to deploy calorie counters, no need for a problematic six to eight meals a day, and certainly no strange or amusing workout exercises required. If you pair it with the satisfying high-fat keto meals, you enter a scenario where hunger could indeed become an outsider.

As another good spin-off, having to re-learn what real hunger feels like still arrives. We get incidents of hunger on a carb-rich diet, and our blood sugar levels appear to fluctuate dramatically as our cells become increasingly desensitized by insulin. The propensity to feed on impulse is often enhanced by sugar, which can really ruin any diet! We will also have to wake up and take care anytime we feel those hunger pangs when we cut back on carbohydrates and ratchet up on the fats, so that will be proper signs that the body needs extra energy.

Chapter 5- Benefits of Ketogenic Diet

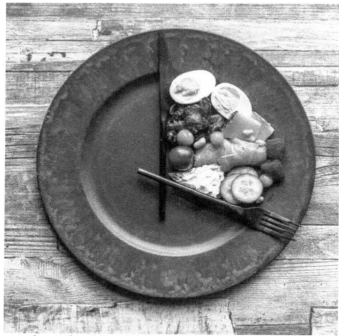

All in all, the straightforward method to the keto diet has inspired individuals to engage with it, resulting in many variants of the keto diet that are available. The keto diet method has been one of the most attempted regimes, and in the last few years, it has grown tremendously in prominence.

Although the key advantage of Keto is successful weight loss, metabolic boosting and hunger control, such advantages include the following-

1. Acne may be decreased by the keto diet since glucose restriction can tip the dynamics of bacteria in the intestine that influences the face.
2. It is known to deter and cure some cancers and, in addition to radiation and chemotherapy, is seen as a supportive medication since it allows cancer cells to undergo additional oxidative stress, allowing them to die.
3. This diet provides your body with a better and healthy source of energy and thus will make you feel more energetic throughout the day.
4. A reduction in cholesterol is caused by keto diets, and the presence of healthy cholesterol is improved.
5. The brain and nerve cells are reinforced and preserved. In addition, it is understood to manage diseases such as Alzheimer's, Parkinson's etc.
6. Many types of research have shown that the keto diet helps to lower down the low-density lipoproteins or the bad cholesterol over time and have been shown to eliminate diseases such as type 2 diabetes.
7. It aids in losing weight as the body burns down the fat as the prior energy source, and one will primarily be using the fat stored in the body as an energy source while in a fasting mode.
8. A Keto diet has been shown to improve cholesterol levels and triglyceride levels most associated with arterial buildup.
9. Known for managing epilepsy-like disorders, Ovarian polycystic disease, etc.

10. The ketogenic diet promises many keto advantages, but a true effort is to initiate the keto diet. It is a restrictive diet that seeks to reduce one's carb consumption to about 50 grams a day, so visiting a dietician to work out and modify the diet according to one's needs is advantageous.

Chapter 6- The 15-day Meal Plan with Low-Carb Recipes that fit the Intermittent Fasting Diet

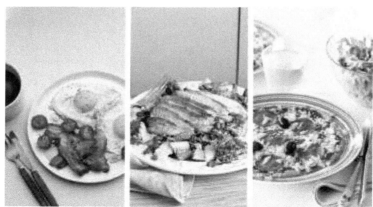

Eating Keto involves limiting the net carb consumption such that energy and ketones are generated by your body metabolizing fat. For many, this means reducing net carbs to 20 grams a day.

The keto diet could be perfect for you if you are trying to optimize advantages such as curing type 2 diabetes or if you want to lose the extra kilos

A more balanced low-carb diet could be a safer option for you if you want more carbohydrates in your diet and if you don't have type 2 diabetes or have a lot of weight to lose. It may be better to adopt mild low carb, but it may also be less successful than Keto, suggesting you may get more modest outcomes.

Day 1

Breakfast- Scrambled eggs

Lunch-Bacon and Zucchini Noodles Salad

Dinner- Spinach Soup

Day 2

Breakfast- Keto Frittata

Lunch-Keto Roasted Pepper and Cauliflower

Dinner-Buffalo Blue Cheese Chicken Wedges

Day 3

Breakfast- Breakfast Bowl

Lunch-Lunch Tacos

Dinner-Lemon Dill Trout

Day 4

Breakfast- Poached Eggs

Lunch-Simple Pizza Rolls

Dinner-Special Fish Pie

Day 5

Breakfast- Bright Morning Smoothie

Lunch-Lunch Stuffed Peppers

Dinner-Cauliflower Bread Garlic Sticks

Day 6

Breakfast-Pumpkin Muffins

Lunch-Lunch Stuffed Peppers

Dinner- Buffalo Blue Cheese Chicken Wedges

Day 7

Breakfast- Keto Breakfast Mix

Lunch-Lunch Caesar Salad

Dinner-Sage N Orange Breast of Duck

Day 8

Breakfast-Pumpkin Pie Spiced Latte

Lunch-Keto Roasted Pepper and Cauliflower

Dinner- Salmon with Caper Sauce

Day 9

Breakfast- Strawberry Protein Smoothie

Lunch-Keto Slow Cooker Buffalo Chicken Soup

Dinner-Cauliflower Bread Garlic Sticks

Day 10

Breakfast-Delicious Eggs and Sausages

Lunch-Special Lunch Burgers

Dinner-Tossed Brussel Sprout Salad

Day 11

Breakfast-Bright Morning Smoothie

Lunch-Keto Lunch Jambalaya

Dinner- Spinach Soup

Day 12

Breakfast-Keto Frittata

Lunch-Lunch Tacos

Dinner-Special Fish Pie

Day 13

Breakfast-Feta and Asparagus Delight

Lunch-Keta Chicken Enchilada Soup

Dinner-Bok Choy Stir Fry

Day 14

Breakfast-Scrambled Eggs

Lunch- Simple Pizza Rolls

Dinner- Lemon Dill Trout

Day 15

Breakfast-Strawberry Protein Smoothie

Lunch-Bacon and Zucchini Noodles Salad

Dinner-Spinach Soup

The list of food items in this meal plan is not exhaustive. You can change the menu as per the availability of the products.

If you wish to avoid your breakfast or any other meal in order to practice fasting, then you are supposed to keep drinking water in that period of time and also make sure that you take multivitamins prescribed by a physician.

Following provided is a list of foods that you can take while on intermittent fasting inspired keto diet-

1. Vegetables
2. Proteins
3. Oil and good fats
4. Beverages
5. Seeds and nuts
6. Diary

The list of foods provided under are to be completely avoided or should be taken in a minimal amount-

1. Processed Foods
2. Artificial Sweeteners
3. Alcohol
4. Milk
5. Refined fats
6. Legumes
7. Soy Products
8. Grains

9.

Chapter 7- Breakfast Recipes

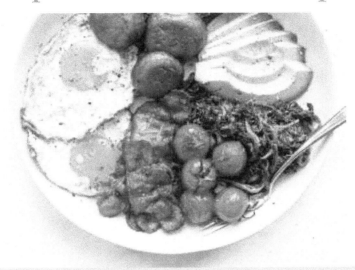

7.1 Delicious Poached Eggs

Ready in about 45 minutes | Servings-4 | Difficulty- Easy

Ingredients

- Three minced garlic cloves
- One tablespoon of ghee
- One chopped white onion
- One chopped Serrano pepper
- Salt and black pepper to the taste
- One chopped red bell pepper
- Three chopped tomatoes
- One teaspoon of paprika
- One teaspoon of cumin
- A quarter teaspoon of chili powder
- One tablespoon of chopped cilantro
- Six eggs

Instructions

1. Heat the pan over medium heat with the ghee, add the onion, stir and cook and stir for ten minutes.
2. Add the garlic and Serrano pepper, stir and cook over medium heat for a minute.
3. Add red bell pepper and cook for 10 minutes, stirring and cooking.
4. Add the tomatoes, pepper, salt, chili powder, paprika and cumin, stir and cook for 10 minutes.
5. In the pan, crack the eggs, season them with pepper and salt, cover the pan and cook for another 6 minutes.
6. In the end, sprinkle with cilantro and serve.

7.2 Delicious Eggs and Sausages

Ready in about 45 minutes | Servings-6 | Difficulty- Easy

Ingredient

- Five tablespoons of ghee
- Twelve eggs
- Salt and black pepper as per taste
- One of torn spinach
- Twelve slices of ham
- Two chopped sausages
- One chopped yellow onion
- One chopped red bell pepper

Instructions

1. Heat a saucepan over medium heat with one tablespoon of ghee, add the onion and sausages, stir and cook for five minutes.
2. Add the bell pepper, pepper and salt, stir and cook for an additional three minutes and place in a bowl.
3. Melt and divide the rest of the ghee into 1two cups of cake molds.
4. In each cupcake mold, add a slice of ham, divide each spinach and then the sausage mix.
5. Break an egg on top, place everything in the oven and bake for 20 minutes at 425 ° Fahrenheit
6. Before serving, leave your cupcakes to cool down a bit.

7.3 Delicious Breakfast Bowl

Ready in about 30 minutes | Servings-1 | Difficulty- Easy

Ingredients

- Four ounces of ground beef
- One chopped yellow onion
- Eight sliced mushrooms
- Salt and black pepper as per taste
- Two whisked eggs
- One tablespoon of coconut oil
- Half a teaspoon of teaspoon smoked paprika
- One avocado, pitted, peeled and chopped
- Twelve pitted and sliced black olives

Instructions

1. Heat a saucepan over medium heat with the coconut oil, add the onions, mushrooms, pepper and salt, stir and cook for five minutes.
2. Add the beef and paprika, stir, cook and transfer to a bowl for 10 minutes.
3. Over medium heat, heat the pan again, add the eggs, some pepper and salt and scramble.
4. Put the beef mix back in the pan and stir.
5. Add the olives and avocado, stir, and cook over medium heat for a minute
6. Transfer and serve in a bowl.

7.4 Keto Breakfast Mix

Ready in about 20 minutes | Servings-2 | Difficulty- Easy

Ingredients

- Five tablespoons of unsweetened coconut flakes
- Seven tablespoons of Hemp seeds
- Five tablespoons of Ground Flaxseed
- Two tablespoons of ground Sesame
- Two tablespoons of unsweetened cocoa, dark
- Two tablespoons of Psyllium husk

Instructions:

1. Grind the sesame and the flaxseed. Ensure that you only grind the sesame seeds for a short time.
2. In a jar, mix all the ingredients and shake them well.
3. Keep refrigerated until ready for consumption.
4. Serve softened with black coffee or still water and, if you want to increase your fat intake, add coconut oil. It also combines well with cream or with cheese from mascarpone.

7.5 Pumpkin Pie Keto Spiced Latte

Ready in about 20 minutes | Servings-2 | Difficulty- Easy

Ingredients

- Two cups of strong and freshly brewed coffee
- One cup of Coconut Milk
- A quarter cup of Pumpkin Puree
- Half teaspoon of Cinnamon
- One teaspoon of Vanilla Extract
- Two teaspoons of Pumpkin Pie Spice Blend
- 15 drops of Liquid Stevia
- Two tablespoons of Butter
- Two tablespoons of Heavy Whipping Cream

Instructions

1. Cook the pumpkin, butter, milk and spices over medium-low flame,
2. Add two cups of solid coffee and blend together until bubbling.
3. Remove from the stove, apply cream and stevia, and then whisk together with an electric mixer.
4. Top with whipped cream and enjoy.

7.6 Keto Frittata

Ready in about one hour 10 minutes | Servings-4 | Difficulty- Moderate

Ingredients

- Nine ounces of spinach
- Twelve eggs
- One ounce of pepperoni
- One teaspoon of minced garlic

- Salt and black pepper to the taste
- Five ounces of shredded mozzarella
- Half cup of grated parmesan
- Half cup of ricotta cheese
- Four tablespoons of olive oil
- A pinch of nutmeg

Instructions

1. Squeeze out the spinach liquid and put it in a bowl.
2. Mix the eggs with the salt, nutmeg, pepper, and garlic in another bowl and whisk well.
3. Add the spinach, ricotta and parmesan and whisk well.
4. Pour this into a saucepan, sprinkle on top with mozzarella and pepperoni, place in the oven and bake for 45 minutes at 375 ° Fahrenheit.
5. Leave the frittata for a few minutes to cool down before serving.

7.7 Keto Fall Pumpkin Spiced French Toast

Ready in about 20 minutes | Servings-2 | Difficulty- Easy

Ingredients

- Four slices of Pumpkin Bread
- One large Egg
- Two tablespoons of cream
- Half teaspoon of Vanilla Extract
- 1/8 teaspoon of Orange Extract
- A quarter teaspoon of Pumpkin Pie Spice
- Two tablespoons of butter

Instructions

Cook the pumpkin, butter, milk and spices over a medium-low flame.

Add two cups of solid coffee and blend together until bubbling.

Remove from the stove, apply cream and stevia, and then whisk together with an electric mixer.

Top with whipped cream and serve.

7.8 Scrambled Eggs

Ready in about 20 minutes | Servings-1 | Difficulty- Easy

Ingredients

- Four chopped bell mushrooms
- Three whisked eggs
- Salt and black pepper to the taste
- Two chopped ham slices
- A quarter cup of chopped red bell pepper
- Half cup of chopped spinach
- One tablespoon of coconut oil

Instructions

Heat a saucepan over medium heat with half the oil, add the mushrooms, spinach, bell pepper and ham, stir and simmer for four minutes.

Heat up another pan over medium heat with the rest of the oil, add the eggs and scramble them.

Stir in the vegetables and ham, pepper and salt, stir, simmer and cook for one minute and then serve.

7.9 Feta and Asparagus Delight

Ready in about 35 minutes | Servings-2 | Difficulty- Easy

Ingredients

- Twelve asparagus spears
- One tablespoon of olive oil
- Two chopped green onions
- One minced garlic clove
- Six eggs
- Salt and black pepper to the taste
- Half cup of feta cheese

Instructions

1. Heat a pan over medium heat with some water, add asparagus, stir for eight minutes, drain well, chop two spears and reserve the remainder.
2. Over medium heat, heat a pan with the oil, add the garlic, onions and chopped asparagus, stir and cook for five minutes.
3. Add salt, pepper and eggs, stir, cover and cook for five minutes.
4. On top of your frittata, arrange the whole asparagus, sprinkle with cheese, place in the oven at 350 ° F and bake for nine minutes.
5. Divide and serve between plates.

7.10 Eggs Baked in Avocados

Ready in about 30 minutes | Servings-4 | Difficulty- Easy

Ingredients

- Two avocados, cut in halves and pitted
- Four eggs
- Salt and black pepper to the taste
- One tablespoon of chopped chives

Instructions

1. Scoop some of the avocado halves with some flesh and assemble them in a baking dish.
2. In each avocado, crack an egg, season with pepper and salt, place them at 425 degrees F in the oven and bake for 20 minutes.
3. In the end, sprinkle the chives and serve them for breakfast.

Chapter 8- Lunch Recipes

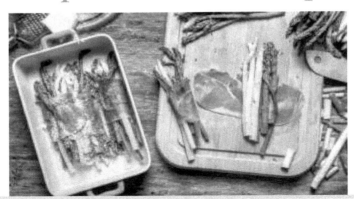

8.1 Lunch Caesar Salad

Ready in about 10 minutes | Servings-2 | Difficulty- Easy

Ingredients

- One pitted, peeled and sliced avocado
- Salt and black pepper to the taste
- Three tablespoons of creamy Caesar dressing
- One cup of cooked and crumbled bacon
- One grilled and shredded chicken breast

Instructions

1. Mix the avocado with the chicken breast and bacon in a salad bowl and stir.
2. Add salt and pepper, Caesar dressing, toss to coat, split into two bowls and serve.

8.2 Keto Lunch Jambalaya

Ready in about 40 minutes | Servings-2 | Difficulty- Moderate

Ingredients

- One medium cauliflower
- One coarsely chopped green pepper
- Two stalks of coarsely chopped celery
- One diced small onion
- Two minced cloves of garlic
- Three cubed boneless chicken breasts
- Eight ounces of sliced smoked sausage
- Eight ounces of ham, cubed
- Fourteen and a half ounce can of diced tomatoes, undrained
- Eight ounce can of tomato sauce
- Three teaspoons of Cajun Seasoning
- Salt and pepper according to taste
- Cooking oil

Instructions

1. Heat two tablespoons of oil in an 8-quart Dutch oven or skillet.
2. On a medium-high flame, sauté the peppers, garlic, chicken, celery, onion and Cajun seasoning until the chicken is almost cooked.
3. Add the cauliflower, ham and sausage. Mix thoroughly.
4. Add the tomato sauce and tomatoes to the mix. Bring it to a simmer, and then turn it back to low.
5. Cover until the cauliflower is moist but not mushy, and cook for around twenty minutes.
6. Season with salt and pepper and then serve after removing from heat.

8.3 Lunch Tacos

Ready in about 40 minutes | Servings-3 | Difficulty- Moderate

Ingredients

- Two cups of grated cheddar cheese
- One small pitted, peeled and chopped avocado
- One cup of cooked favorite taco meat
- Two teaspoons of sriracha sauce
- A quarter cup of chopped tomatoes
- Cooking spray
- Salt and black pepper as per taste

Instructions

1. Spray on a lined baking dish with some cooking oil.
2. Cover on the baking sheet with cheddar cheese, put in the oven at 400 degrees F, and bake for 15 minutes.
3. Spread the taco meat over the cheese and cook for a further 10 minutes.
4. Meanwhile, combine the avocado with tomatoes, sriracha, salt and pepper in a bowl and swirl.
5. Spread this over the layers of taco and cheddar, let the tacos cool down a little, use a pizza slicer to slice and serve for lunch.

8.4 Keto Chicken Enchilada Soup

Ready in about 40 minutes | Servings-3 | Difficulty- Moderate

Ingredients

- Six oz. Shredded chicken
- Two teaspoons of Cumin
- One teaspoon of Oregano
- One teaspoon of Chili Powder
- Half teaspoon of Cayenne Pepper
- Half cup of chopped cilantro
- Half medium Lime, juiced
- three tablespoons of Olive Oil
- Three stalks of diced Celery
- One medium diced Red Bell Pepper, diced
- Two teaspoons of garlic, minced

- Four cups of Chicken Broth
- One cup of Diced Tomatoes
- Eight oz. of Cream Cheese

Instructions

1. Heat the oil in a pan and add the celery and pepper. Add the tomatoes and cook for 2-3 minutes once the celery is soft.
2. Add the spices to the pan and mix well.
3. Add the chicken broth and the cilantro to the mixture, boil, and then reduce to low for 20 minutes to simmer.
4. Then add the cream cheese and bring it back to the boil. Once it has cooked, reduce the heat to low and cover and cook for 25 minutes.
5. Scrap the chicken and add it to the pot, then top it with half the lime juice.
6. Mix together everything.
7. Serve with coriander, sour cream or shredded cheese.

8.5 Simple Pizza Rolls

Ready in about 40 minutes | Servings-6 | Difficulty- Moderate

Ingredients

- A quarter cups of chopped mixed red and green bell peppers
- Two cups of shredded mozzarella cheese
- One teaspoon of pizza seasoning
- Two tablespoons of chopped onion
- One chopped tomato
- Salt and black pepper to the taste
- A quarter cups of pizza sauce
- Half cup of crumbled and cooked sausage

Instructions

1. On a lined and lightly oiled baking dish, spread mozzarella cheese, sprinkle pizza seasoning on top, put at 400 °F in the oven and bake for 20 minutes.
2. Spread the sausage, onion, tomatoes and bell pepper all over and drizzle the tomato sauce at the top. Taking the pizza crust out of the oven.
3. Place them back in the oven and bake for ten more minutes.
4. Take the pizza from the oven, leave it aside for a few minutes, break it into six pieces, roll each slice and eat it for lunch.

8.6 Lunch Stuffed Peppers

Ready in about 50 minutes | Servings-4 | Difficulty- Moderate

Ingredients

- Four big banana peppers cut into halves lengthwise
- One tablespoon of ghee
- Salt and black pepper to the taste
- Half teaspoon of herbs de Provence
- One pound of chopped sweet sausage
- Three tablespoons of chopped yellow onions
- Some marinara sauce

- A drizzle of olive oil

Instructions

1. Season the banana peppers with pepper and salt, drizzle with the oil, rub well and bake for 20 minutes in the oven at 325 ° F.
2. Meanwhile, over medium, prepare, heat a skillet, add the pieces of sausage, mix and cook for 5 minutes.
3. Combine the onion, herbs, salt, pepper and ghee, mix well and simmer for 5 minutes.
4. Take the peppers out of the oven, load them with the sausage mix, place them in a dish that is oven-proof, drizzle them with the marinara sauce, placed them back in the oven and bake for another 10 minutes.
5. Serve and enjoy.

8.7 Special Lunch Burgers

Ready in about 35 minutes | Servings-8 | Difficulty- Moderate

Ingredients

- One pound ground brisket
- One pound ground beef
- Salt and black pepper as per taste
- Eight butter slices
- One tablespoon of minced garlic
- One tablespoon of Italian seasoning
- Two tablespoons of mayonnaise
- One tablespoon of ghee
- Two tablespoons of olive oil
- One chopped yellow onion
- One tablespoon of water

Instructions

1. Mix the beef, pepper, salt, Italian herbs, mayo and garlic with the brisket in a bowl and stir well.
2. Form 8 patties into each one to create a pocket.
3. With butter-slices, stuff each burger and seal it.
4. Over medium pressure, heat the pan with the oil, add the onions, stir and simmer for 2 minutes.
5. Apply the water, swirl and pick them up in the pan corner.
6. Put the burgers with the onions in the pan and cook them for ten minutes over moderate flame.
7. Flip them over, apply the ghee, and simmer for ten more minutes.
8. Break the burgers into buns and place them on top of caramelized onions.

8.8 Keto Roasted Pepper and Cauliflower

Ready in about 50 minutes | Servings-4 | Difficulty- Moderate

Ingredients

- Two halved and de-seeded Red Bell Peppers
- Half head of cauliflower cut into florets

- Two tablespoons of Duck Fat
- Three medium diced green Onions
- Three cups of Chicken Broth
- Half cup Heavy Cream
- Four tablespoons of Duck Fat
- Salt and pepper as per taste
- One teaspoon of Garlic Powder
- One teaspoon of Dried Thyme
- One teaspoon of Smoked Paprika
- A quarter teaspoon of Red Pepper Flakes
- Four oz. Goat Cheese

Instructions

1. Preheat the oven to 400 °F

Clean, de-seed, and half-slice the peppers

Broil until the flesh is burnt and blackened for about 10-15 minutes.

Place in a container with a cover to steam when finished cooking cauliflower.

Sprinkle two tablespoons of melted duck fat, pepper and salt into sliced cauliflower florets.

Cook for 30-35 minutes in the oven.

Pick off the skins of the peppers by gently peeling them off.

Heat Four tablespoons of duck fat in a pot and add the diced green onion.

To toast, apply seasonings to the plate, then add red pepper, chicken broth, and cauliflower to the skillet.

For 10-20 minutes, let this boil.

Bring the mixture to an immersion blender. Make sure that it emulsifies both fats.

Then apply the cream and combine.

Serve with some bacon and goats' cheese. Add thyme and green onion to garnish.

8.9 Bacon and Zucchini Noodles Salad

Ready in about 10 minutes | Servings-2 | Difficulty- Easy

Ingredients

- One cup of baby spinach
- Four cups of zucchini noodles
- 1/3 cups of crumbled bleu cheese
- 1/3 cups of thick cheese dressing
- Half cup of cooked and crumbled bacon
- Black pepper as per taste

Instructions

1. Mix the spinach with the bacon, zucchini noodles and the bleu cheese in a salad dish, and toss.
2. Apply the black pepper and cheese dressing as per taste, toss well to cover, distribute into two bowls and eat.

8.10 Keto Slow Cooker Buffalo Chicken Soup

Ready in about 6 hours and 20 minutes | Servings-2 | Difficulty- Hard

Ingredients

- Three Chicken Thighs, de-boned and sliced
- One teaspoon of Onion Powder
- One teaspoon of Garlic Powder
- Half teaspoon Celery Seed
- A quarter cup of butter
- Half cup of Frank's Hot Sauce
- Three cups of Beef Broth
- One cup of Heavy Cream
- Two oz. Cream Cheese
- A quarter teaspoon of Xanthan Gum
- Salt and pepper as per taste

Instructions

1. Begin by de-boning the chicken thighs, break the chicken into chunks and place the remainder of the ingredients in a slow cooker in the crockpot with the exception of cream, cheese, and xanthan gum.
2. Set a low, slow cooker for 6 hours (or a high one for 3 hours) and cook fully.
3. Remove the chicken from the slow cooker until it is done, and shred it with a fork.
4. Using the slow cooker to combine cream, cheese, and xanthan gum. Combine it all together
5. Transfer the chicken to the slow cooker and blend.
6. Season it with salt, pepper, and hot sauce. Serve.

Chapter 9- Dinner Recipes

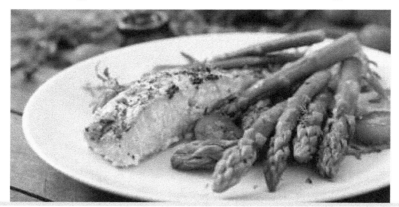

9.1 Buffalo Blue Cheese Chicken Wedges

Ready in about 40 minutes | Servings-2 | Difficulty-Moderate

Ingredients

- One head of lettuce
- Bleu cheese dressing
- Two tablespoons of crumbled blue cheese
- Four strips of bacon
- Two boneless chicken breasts
- 3/4 cup of any buffalo sauce

Instructions

1. Boil a big pot of salted water.
2. Add two chicken breasts to the water and simmer for 30 minutes, or until the internal temperature of the chicken reaches 180 °C.
3. Let the chicken rest for 10 minutes to cool.
4. Take apart the chicken into strips using a fork.
5. Cook and cool bacon strips, crumble reserve,
6. Merge the scrapped chicken and buffalo sauce over medium heat, then mix until warm.
7. Break the lettuce into wedges and apply the appropriate amount of blue cheese dressing to it.
8. Add crumbles of blue cheese.
9. Add the chicken-pulled buffalo.
10. Cover with more crumbles of blue cheese and fried crumbled bacon.
11. Serve.

9.2 Cauliflower Bread Garlic sticks

Ready in about 55 minutes | Servings-2 | Difficulty-Moderate

Ingredients

- Two cups of cauliflower rice
- One tablespoon of organic butter
- Three teaspoons of minced garlic

- A quarter teaspoon of red pepper flakes
- Half teaspoon of Italian seasoning
- 1/8 teaspoon of kosher salt
- One cup of shredded mozzarella cheese
- One egg
- One cup of grated parmesan cheese

Instructions

1. Preheat the oven to 350° F.
2. Sauté the red pepper flakes and garlic for nearly three minutes and transfer to a bowl of cooked cauliflower. Melt the butter in a small skillet over low heat.
3. Mix the Italian seasoning and salt together.
4. Afterward, refrigerate for 10 minutes.
5. Add the mozzarella cheese and egg to the cauliflower mixture until slightly cooled.
6. A creamy paste in a thin layer lined with parchment paper on a thinly oiled 9-9 baking dish.
7. Bake for thirty minutes.
8. Remove from the oven and finish with a little more parmesan and mozzarella cheese.
9. Put them back in the oven and cook for an extra 8 minutes.
10. Remove from the oven and slice into sticks of the appropriate duration.

9.3 Tasty Baked Fish

Ready in about 40 minutes | Servings-4 | Difficulty-Moderate

Ingredients

- One pound of haddock
- Three teaspoons of water
- Two tablespoons of lemon juice
- Salt and black pepper as per taste
- Two tablespoons of mayonnaise
- One teaspoon of dill weed
- Cooking spray
- A pinch of old bay seasoning

Instructions

1. With some cooking oil, spray a baking dish.
2. Apply the lemon juice, fish and water and toss to cover a little bit.
3. Apply salt, pepper, seasoning with old bay and dill weed and mix again.
4. Add mayonnaise and spread evenly.
5. Place it at 350 ° F in the oven and bake for thirty minutes.
6. Split and serve on a plate.

9.4 Spinach Soup

Ready in about 25 minutes | Servings-8 | Difficulty-Easy

Ingredients

- Two tablespoons of ghee
- Twenty ounces of chopped spinach
- One teaspoon of minced garlic
- Salt and black pepper as per taste

- Forty-five ounces of chicken stock
- Half teaspoons of nutmeg, ground
- Two cups of heavy cream
- One chopped yellow onion

Instructions

1. Heat a pot over medium heat with the ghee, add the onion, stir and simmer for 4 minutes.
2. Stir in the garlic, stir and simmer for a minute.
3. Add spinach and stock and simmer for 5 minutes.
4. Blend the broth with an immersion mixer and reheat the soup.
5. Stir in pepper, nutmeg, salt, and cream, stir and simmer for a further 5 minutes.
6. Ladle it into cups and serve.

9.5 Tossed Brussel Sprout Salad

Ready in about 30 minutes | Servings-2 | Difficulty-Easy

Ingredients

- Six Brussels sprouts
- Half teaspoon of apple cider vinegar
- One teaspoon of olive/grapeseed oil
- A quarter teaspoon of salt
- A quarter teaspoon of pepper
- One tablespoon of freshly grated parmesan

Instructions

1. Break and clean Brussels sprouts in half lengthwise, root on, then cut thin slices through them in the opposite direction.
2. Cut the roots and remove them until chopped.
3. Toss the apple cider, oil, pepper and salt together.
4. Sprinkle, blend and eat with your parmesan cheese.

9.6 Special Fish Pie

Ready in about One hour 20 minutes | Servings-6 | Difficulty-Moderate

Ingredients

- One chopped red onion
- Two skinless and medium sliced salmon fillets
- Two skinless and medium sliced mackerel fillets
- Three medium sliced haddock fillets
- Two bay leaves
- A quarter cup and two tablespoons of ghee
- One cauliflower head, florets separated
- Four eggs
- Four cloves
- One cup of whipping cream
- Half cup of water
- A pinch of nutmeg
- One teaspoon of Dijon mustard
- One and a half cup of shredded cheddar cheese

- A handful of chopped parsley
- Salt and black pepper as per taste
- Four tablespoons of chopped chives

Instructions

1. In a saucepan, place some water, add some salt, bring to a boil over medium heat, add the eggs, simmer for ten minutes, heat off, drain, cool, peel and break into quarters.
2. Place the water in another kettle, bring it to a boil, add the florets of cauliflower, simmer for 10 minutes, rinse, add a quarter of a cup of ghee, add it to the mixer, blend properly, and place it in a bowl.
3. Add the cream and half a cup of water to a saucepan, add the fish, toss and cover over medium heat.
4. Put to a boil, reduce heat to a minimum, and steam for 10 minutes. Put the cloves, onion, and bay leave.
5. Take the heat off, put the fish and set it aside in a baking dish.
6. Heat the saucepan with the fish, add the nutmeg, combine and simmer for 5 minutes.
7. Remove from the oven, discard the bay leaves and cloves and blend well with one cup of cheddar cheese and two tablespoons of ghee.
8. On top of the fish, set the egg quarters in the baking dish.
9. Sprinkle with cream and cheese sauce on top of the remaining cheddar cheese, chives and parsley, cover with cauliflower mash, sprinkle with the remaining cheddar cheese, and place in the oven for 30 minutes at 400 ° F.
10. Leave the pie until it is about to slice and serve, to cool down a little.

9.7 Lemon Dill Trout

Ready in about 20 minutes | Servings-4 | Difficulty-Easy

Ingredients

- Two pounds of pan-dressed trout (or other small fish), fresh or frozen
- One and a half teaspoons of salt
- A quarter teaspoon of pepper
- Half cup of butter or margarine
- Two tablespoons of dill weed
- Three tablespoons of lemon juice

Instructions

1. Cut fish lengthwise and season its inside with pepper and salt.
2. With melted butter and dill weed, prepare a frying pan.
3. For about two to three minutes per side, fry the fish flesh side down.
4. Remove the fish.
5. Add lemon juice to butter and dill to create a sauce.
6. Serve the fish and sauce together.

9.8 Sage N Orange Breast of Duck

Ready in about 20 minutes | Servings-4 | Difficulty-Easy

Ingredients

- Six oz. Duck Breast (~6 oz.)
- Two tablespoons of Butter
- One tablespoon of Heavy Cream
- One tablespoon of Swerve
- Half teaspoon of Orange Extract
- A quarter teaspoon of Sage
- One cup of spinach

Instructions

1. Score the duck skin on top of the breast and season with pepper and salt.
2. Brown butter in a saucepan over medium-low heat, and swerve.
3. Add the extract of sage and orange and cook until it is deep orangey in color.
4. Sear duck breasts for few minutes until nicely crunchy.
5. Flip the Breast of the Duck.
6. Add the orange and sage butter to the heavy cream and pour it over the duck.
7. Cook until finished.
8. In the pan that you used to make the sauce, add the spinach and serve with the duck.

9.9 Salmon with Caper Sauce

Ready in about 30 minutes | Servings-3 | Difficulty-Easy

Ingredients

- Three salmon fillets
- Salt and black pepper as per taste
- One tablespoon of olive oil
- One tablespoon of Italian seasoning
- Two tablespoons of capers
- Three tablespoons of lemon juice
- Four minced garlic cloves
- Two tablespoons of ghee

Instructions

1. Heat the olive oil pan over medium heat, add the skin of the fish fillets side by side, season with pepper salt and Italian seasoning, cook for two minutes, toss and cook for another two minutes, remove from heat, cover and leave aside for 15 minutes.
2. Put the fish on a plate and leave it aside.
3. Over medium heat, heat the same pan, add the capers, garlic and lemon juice, stir and cook for two minutes.
4. Remove the heat from the pan, add ghee and stir very well.
5. Put the fish back in the pan and toss with the sauce to coat.
6. Divide and serve on plates.

9.10 Bok Choy Stir Fry

Ready in about 20 minutes | Servings-2 | Difficulty-Easy

Ingredients

- Two minced garlic cloves
- Two cups of chopped bok choy
- Two chopped bacon slices
- Salt and black pepper to the taste
- A drizzle of avocado oil

Instructions

1. Heat a pan over medium heat with the oil, add the bacon, stir and brown until crunchy, move to paper towels and drain the oil.
2. Return the saucepan to medium heat, stir in the garlic and bok choy, and cook for 4 minutes.
3. Stir in salt, pepper and bacon, stir, cook for another 1 minute, divide among plates and serve.

Chapter 10- Appetizer and Snacks Recipes

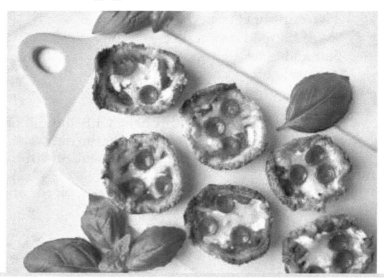

10.1 Cheeseburger Muffins

Ready in about 40 minutes | Servings-9 | Difficulty-Easy

Ingredients

- Half cups of flaxseed meal
- Half cups of almond flour
- Salt and black pepper to the taste
- Two eggs
- One teaspoon of baking powder
- A quarter cups of sour cream

For the filling

- Half teaspoons of onion powder
- Sixteen ounces of ground beef
- Salt and black pepper to the taste
- Two tablespoons of tomato paste
- Half teaspoons of garlic powder
- Half cups of grated cheddar cheese
- Two tablespoons of mustard

Instructions

1. Mix the almond flour with the flaxseed meal, pepper, salt and baking powder in a bowl and whisk together.
2. Add the sour cream and eggs and stir very well.
3. Divide it into a greased muffin pan and use your fingers to press well.
4. Over medium-high heat, heat a pan, add beef, stir and brown for a couple of minutes.
5. Stir well and add pepper, salt, garlic powder, onion powder and tomato paste.
6. Cook for an additional 5 minutes and take the heat off.
7. Fill the crusts with this mixture, place them in the oven at 350 degrees F and bake for fifteen minutes
8. Spread the cheese on top, put it in the oven again and cook the muffins for another 5 minutes.

9. Serve with mustard and your preferred toppings.

10.2 Pesto Crackers

Ready in about 30 minutes | Servings-6 | Difficulty-Easy

Ingredients

- Half teaspoons of baking powder
- Salt and black pepper to the taste
- One and a quarter cups of almond flour
- A quarter teaspoon of basil, dried
- One minced garlic clove
- Two tablespoons of basil pesto
- A pinch of cayenne pepper
- Three tablespoons of ghee

Instructions

1. Mix the pepper, salt, almond flour and baking powder together in a bowl.
2. Stir in the garlic, basil and cayenne.
3. Add whisk the pesto.
4. Also, add ghee and with your finger, mix your dough.
5. Spread this dough on a baking sheet and bake it at 325 degrees F in the oven for 17 minutes.
6. Leave your crackers aside to cool down, cut them and serve.

10.3 Tomato Tarts

Ready in about One hour and 20 minutes | Servings-4 | Difficulty-Easy

Ingredients

- A quarter cups of olive oil
- Two sliced tomatoes
- Salt and black pepper to the taste

For the base

- Five tablespoons of ghee
- One tablespoon psyllium husk
- Half cups of almond flour
- Two tablespoons of coconut flour
- A pinch of salt

For the filling

- Two teaspoons of minced garlic
- Three teaspoons of chopped thyme
- Two tablespoons of olive oil
- Three ounces of crumbled goat cheese
- One small thinly sliced onion

Instructions

1. On a lined baking sheet, spread the tomato slices, season with pepper and salt, drizzle with a quarter of a cup of olive oil, place in the oven at 425 degrees F and bake for 40 minutes.
2. Meanwhile, mix psyllium husk with almond flour, coconut flour, pepper, salt and cold butter in your food processor and stir until you've got your dough.
3. Divide this dough into cupcake molds of silicone, press well, place it in the oven at 350 degrees F and bake for 20 minutes.
4. Remove the cupcakes from the oven and leave them aside.
5. Also, take slices of tomatoes from the oven and cool them down a bit.
6. On top of the cupcakes, divide the tomato slices.
7. Heat a saucepan over medium-high heat with two tablespoons of olive oil, add the onion, stir and cook for 4 minutes.
8. Add the thyme and garlic, stir, cook for another 1 minute and remove from the heat.
9. Spread the mix over the tomato slices.
10. Sprinkle with the goat cheese, put it back in the oven and cook for five more minutes at 350 degrees F.
11. Arrange and serve on a platter.

10.4 Pepper Nachos

Ready in about 30 minutes | Servings-6 | Difficulty-Easy

Ingredients

- One pound of halved mini bell peppers
- Salt and black pepper as per the taste
- One teaspoon of garlic powder
- One teaspoon of sweet paprika
- Half teaspoons of dried oregano
- A quarter teaspoon of red pepper flakes
- One pound of ground beef meat
- One and a half cups of shredded cheddar cheese
- One tablespoon of chili powder
- One teaspoon of ground cumin
- Half cups of chopped tomato
- Sour cream for serving

Instructions

1. Mix the chili powder, pepper, salt, paprika, oregano, cumin, flakes of pepper and garlic powder in a bowl and stir.
2. Over medium heat, heat a pan, add beef, mix and brown for 10 minutes.
3. Add the mixture of chili powder, stir and take the heat off.
4. On a lined baking sheet, arrange the pepper halves, stuff them with the beef mix, sprinkle the cheese, place in the oven at 400 degrees F and cook for 10 minutes.
5. Remove the peppers from the oven, sprinkle with the tomatoes and divide among the plates and serve with sour cream.

10.5 Pumpkin Muffins

Ready in about One hour 25 minutes | Servings-18 | Difficulty-Easy

Ingredients

- A quarter cups of sunflower seed butter
- 3/4 cups of pumpkin puree
- Two tablespoons of flaxseed meal
- A quarter cups of coconut flour
- Half cup of erythritol
- Half teaspoons of ground nutmeg
- one teaspoon of ground cinnamon
- Half teaspoons of baking soda
- One egg
- Half teaspoons of baking powder
- A pinch of salt

Instructions

1. Mix the butter with the pumpkin puree and egg in a bowl and mix well.
2. Stir well and add coconut flour, flaxseed meal, erythritol, baking powder, baking soda, nutmeg, cinnamon and a pinch of salt.
3. Spoon this into an oiled muffin pan, add in the oven at 350 degrees F and cook for 15 minutes.
4. Let the muffins cool and serve them as a snack.

10.6 Fried Queso

Ready in about One hour 20 minutes | Servings-6 | Difficulty-Easy

Ingredients

- Two ounces of pitted and chopped olives,
- Five ounces of cubed and freeze queso Blanco
- A pinch of red pepper flakes
- One and a half tablespoons of olive oil

Instructions

1. Over medium-high heat, heat a pan with the oil, add cheese cubes and fry until the lower part melts a bit.
2. Flip the spatula cubes and sprinkle on top with black olives.
3. Let the cubes cook a little more, flip and sprinkle with the red flakes of pepper and cook until crispy.
4. Flip, cook until crispy on the other side, then move to a chopping board, cut into tiny blocks, and then serve.

10.7 Tortilla Chips

Ready in about 25 minutes | Servings-6 | Difficulty-Easy

Ingredients

For the tortillas

- Two teaspoons of olive oil
- One cup of flaxseed meal
- Two tablespoons of psyllium husk powder
- A quarter teaspoon of xanthan gum
- One cup of water

- Half teaspoons of curry powder
- Three teaspoons of coconut flour

For the chips

- Six flaxseed tortillas
- Salt and black pepper to the taste
- Three tablespoons of vegetable oil
- Fresh salsa for serving
- Sour cream for serving

Instructions

1. Combine psyllium powder, flaxseed meal, xanthan gum, olive oil curry powder and water in a bowl and mix until an elastic dough is obtained.
2. On a working surface, spread coconut flour.
3. Divide the dough into six pieces, place each portion on the work surface, roll it into a circle and cut it into six pieces each.
4. Over medium-high heat, heat a pan with vegetable oil, add tortilla chips, cook on each side for 2 minutes and transfer to paper towels.
5. Put in a bowl of tortilla chips, season with pepper and salt and serve on the side with sour cream and fresh salsa.

10.8 Jalapeno Balls

Ready in about One hour 20 minutes | Servings-3 | Difficulty-Easy

Ingredients

- Three slices of bacon
- Three ounces of cream cheese
- A quarter teaspoon of onion powder
- Salt and black pepper as per taste
- One chopped jalapeno pepper
- Half teaspoons of dried parsley
- A quarter teaspoon of garlic powder

Instructions

1. Over medium-high heat, heat a skillet, add bacon, cook until crispy, switch to paper towels, remove the fat and crumble.
2. Reserve the pan's bacon fat.
3. Combine the jalapeno pepper, cream cheese, garlic powder and onion, parsley, pepper and salt in a bowl and stir thoroughly.
4. Use this blend to mix bacon crumbles and bacon fat, stir softly, form balls, and serve.

10.9 Maple and Pecan Bars

Ready in about 40 minutes | Servings-12 | Difficulty-Easy

Ingredients

- Half cups of flaxseed meal
- two cups of pecans, toasted and crushed
- one cup of almond flour
- Half cups of coconut oil

- A quarter teaspoon of stevia
- Half cups of coconut, shredded
- A quarter cups of maple syrup
- **For the maple syrup**
- A quarter cups of erythritol
- Two and a quarter teaspoons of coconut oil
- One tablespoon of ghee
- A quarter teaspoon of xanthan gum
- 3/4 cups of water
- Two teaspoons of maple extract
- Half teaspoons of vanilla extract

Instructions

1. Combine ghee with two and a quarter teaspoons of xanthan gum and coconut oil in a heat-proof bowl, stir, put in your oven and heat up for 1 minute.
2. Add the extract of erythritol, water, maple and vanilla, mix well and fire for 1 minute more in the microwave.
3. Mix the flaxseed meal and the coconut and almond flour in a bowl and stir.
4. Add the pecans, and stir them again.
5. Apply a quarter of a cup of maple syrup, stevia, and half a cup of coconut oil, and mix well.
6. Spread this in a baking dish, push well, position it at 350 degrees F in the oven and cook for 25 minutes.
7. To cool off, leave it aside, break into 12 bars and act as a keto snack.

10.10 Broccoli and Cheddar Biscuits

Ready in about One hour 35 minutes | Servings-12 | Difficulty-Easy

Ingredients

- Four cups of broccoli florets
- One and a half cups of almond flour
- One teaspoon of paprika
- Salt and black pepper to the taste
- Two eggs
- A quarter cup of coconut oil
- Two cups of grated cheddar cheese
- One teaspoon of garlic powder
- Half teaspoons of apple cider vinegar
- Half teaspoons of baking soda

Instructions

1. In your food processor, place the broccoli florets, add some pepper and salt and combine well.
2. Mix pepper, salt, paprika, baking soda and garlic powder with almond flour in a bowl and stir.
3. Apply the coconut oil, cheddar cheese, vinegar and eggs and stir.
4. Attach the broccoli and stir some more.
5. Shape Twelve patties, arrange them on a baking sheet, put them at 375 degrees F in the oven and bake for 20 minutes.

6. Switch the broiler in the oven and broil the biscuits for another 5 minutes.
7. Arrange and serve on a platter.

Chapter 11- Dessert Recipes

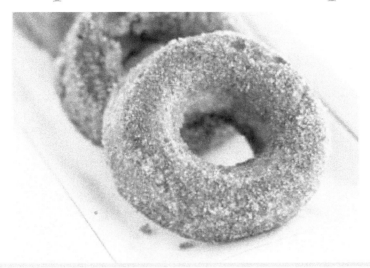

11.1 Chocolate Truffles

Ready in about 20 minutes | Servings-22 | Difficulty-Easy

Ingredients

- One cup of sugar-free chocolate chips
- Two tablespoons of butter
- 2/3 cups of heavy cream
- Two teaspoons of brandy
- Two tablespoons of swerve
- A quarter teaspoon of vanilla extract
- Cocoa powder

Instructions

1. In a fire-proof mug, add heavy cream, swerve, chocolate chips and butter, stir, put in the microwave and heat for 1 minute.
2. Leave for 5 minutes, blend well, and combine with the vanilla and the brandy.
3. Stir again. Set aside for a few hours in the fridge.
4. Shape the truffles using a melon baller, cover them in cocoa powder and then serve them.

11.2 Keto Doughnuts

Ready in about 25 minutes | Servings-24 | Difficulty-Easy

Ingredients

- A quarter cups of erythritol
- A quarter cups of flaxseed meal
- 3/4 cups of almond flour
- One teaspoon of baking powder
- One teaspoon of vanilla extract
- Two eggs
- Three tablespoons of coconut oil

- A quarter cups of coconut milk
- Twenty drops of red food coloring
- A pinch of salt
- One tablespoon of cocoa powder

Instructions

1. Mix together the almond flour, cocoa powder, baking powder, erythritol and salt in a bowl and stir.
2. Mix the coconut oil with vanilla, coconut milk, food coloring and eggs in another bowl and stir.
3. Mix mixtures, use a hand mixer to stir, move to a bag, cut a hole in the bag and shape a baking sheet with 12 doughnuts.
4. Place it in the oven at 350 degrees F and cook for 15 minutes.
5. On a tray, place them and eat them.

11.3 Chocolate Bombs

Ready in about 20 minutes | Servings-12 | Difficulty-Easy

Ingredients

- Ten tablespoons of coconut oil
- Three tablespoons of chopped macadamia nuts
- Two packets of stevia
- Five tablespoons of unsweetened coconut powder
- A pinch of salt

Instructions

1. Place coconut oil in a casserole dish and melt over medium heat.
2. Apply stevia, salt and cocoa powder, mix well and remove from the heat.
3. Spoon this into a tray of candy and store it for a while in the freezer.
4. Sprinkle the macadamia nuts on top and hold them in the refrigerator until served.

11.4 Simple and Delicious Mousse

Ready in about 10 minutes | Servings-12 | Difficulty-Easy

Ingredients

- Eight ounces of mascarpone cheese
- 3/4 teaspoons of vanilla stevia
- One cup of whipping cream
- Half-pint of blueberries
- Half-pint of strawberries

Instructions

1. Combine the whipped cream with mascarpone and stevia in a cup and blend well with your mixer.
2. Assemble twelve glasses with a coating of strawberries and blueberries, then a layer of milk, and so on.
3. Serve cool.

11.5 Strawberry Pie

Ready in about 2 hours and 20 minutes | Servings-12 | Difficulty-Hard

Ingredients

For the filling

- One teaspoon of gelatin
- Eight ounces of cream cheese
- Four ounces of strawberries
- Two tablespoons of water
- Half tablespoon of lemon juice
- A quarter teaspoon of stevia
- Half cups of heavy cream
- Eight ounces of chopped strawberries for serving
- Sixteen ounces of heavy cream for serving

For the crust

- One cup of shredded coconut
- One cup of sunflower seeds
- A quarter cup of butter
- A pinch of salt

Instructions

1. Mix the sunflower seeds with coconut, butter and a pinch of salt in your food processor and stir well.
2. Place this in a greased springform pan and push the bottom well.
3. Heat a skillet over medium heat with the water, add gelatin, mix until it dissolves, remove the heat and leave to cool off.
4. Add it to your food processor, mix and blend well with 4 ounces of cream cheese, lemon juice, strawberries and stevia.
5. Stir well, pour half a cup of heavy cream and scatter over the crust.
6. Before slicing and serving, top with 8 ounces of strawberries and 16 ounces of heavy cream and keep in the refrigerator for 2 hours.

11.6 Keto Cheesecakes

Ready in about 25 minutes | Servings-9 | Difficulty-Easy

Ingredients

For the cheesecakes

- Two tablespoons of butter
- Eight ounces of cream cheese
- Three tablespoons of coffee
- Three eggs
- 1/3 cups of swerve
- One tablespoon of sugar-free caramel syrup

For the frosting

- Three tablespoons of sugar-free caramel syrup

- Three tablespoons of butter
- Eight ounces of soft mascarpone cheese
- Two tablespoons of swerve

Instructions

1. Combine eggs with cream cheese, two tablespoons butter, one tablespoon caramel syrup, coffee, and 1/3 cup swerve in your blender and pulse very well.
2. Spoon this into a pan of cupcakes, place it at 350 degrees F in the oven and cook for 15 minutes.
3. To cool down, leave aside and then keep in the freezer for three hours.
4. Meanwhile, mix three tablespoons butter with three tablespoons caramel syrup, two tablespoons swerve and mascarpone cheese in a bowl and mix well.
5. Spoon the cheesecakes over and serve them.

11.7 Peanut Butter Fudge

Ready in about 2 hours and 15 minutes | Servings-12 | Difficulty-Hard

Ingredients

- One cup of unsweetened peanut butter
- A quarter cups of almond milk
- Two teaspoons of vanilla stevia
- One cup of coconut oil
- A pinch of salt

For the topping

- Two tablespoons of swerve
- Two tablespoons of melted coconut oil
- A quarter cups of cocoa powder

Instructions

1. Combine peanut butter with one cup of coconut oil in a heat-proof bowl, stir and heat in your microwave until it melts.
2. Add stevia, a pinch of salt and almond milk, mix it well and pour into a lined loaf pan.
3. Keep it for 2 hours in the refrigerator and then slice it.
4. Mix two tablespoons of cocoa powder and melted coconut in a bowl and swirl and stir well.
5. Drizzle over your peanut butter fudge with the sauce and serve.

11.8 Chocolate Pie

Ready in about 3 hours and 30 minutes | Servings-10 | Difficulty-Hard

Ingredients

For the filling

- One tablespoon vanilla extract
- Four tablespoons of sour cream
- One teaspoon of vanilla extract
- Four tablespoons of butter
- Sixteen ounces of cream cheese
- Half cup of cut stevia

- Two teaspoons of granulated stevia
- Half cup of cocoa powder
- One cup of whipping cream

For crust

- Half teaspoons of baking powder
- One and a half cups of the almond crust
- A quarter cup of stevia
- A pinch of salt
- One egg
- One and a half teaspoons of vanilla extract
- Three tablespoons of butter
- One teaspoon of butter for the pan

Instructions

1. With one teaspoon of butter, oil a springform pan and leave aside for now.
2. Mix the baking powder with a quarter cup of stevia, almond flour and a pinch of salt in a bowl and stir.
3. Add three tablespoons of butter, one teaspoon of egg, and one and a half teaspoons of vanilla extract, then mix till the time the dough is ready.
4. Press it well into the springform pan, place it at 375 degrees F in the oven and cook it for 11 minutes.
5. Take the pie crust out of the oven, cover it with tin foil and cook for another 8 minutes.
6. Take it out of the oven again and set it aside to cool down.
7. Meanwhile, add sour cream, four tablespoons of butter, one tablespoon of vanilla extract, half a cup of cocoa powder and stevia to the cream cheese in a bowl and mix it well.
8. Mix two teaspoons of stevia and one teaspoon of vanilla extract with the whipping cream in another bowl and stir using your mixer.
9. Combine two mixtures, pour into the pie crust, spread well, place for 3 hours in the refrigerator and serve.

11.9 Raspberry and Coconut Dessert

Ready in about 20 minutes | Servings-12 | Difficulty-Easy

Ingredients

- Half cup of coconut butter
- Half cup of coconut oil
- Half cup of dried raspberries
- A quarter cups of swerve
- Half cup of shredded coconut

Instructions

1. Mix the dried berries in your food processor very well.
2. Heat a pan over medium heat with the butter.
3. Stir in the coconut, oil and swerve, stir and cook for 5 minutes.
4. Pour half of this and spread well into a lined baking pan.
5. Add raspberry powder and also spread.
6. Spread the rest of the butter mix on top and keep it in the fridge for a while.
7. Cut and serve into pieces.

11.10 Vanilla Ice Cream

Ready in about 3 hours 20 minutes | Servings-6 | Difficulty-Hard

Ingredients

- Four eggs, yolks and whites separated
- A quarter teaspoon of cream of tartar
- Half cups of swerve
- One tablespoon of vanilla extract
- One and a quarter cups of heavy whipping cream

Instructions

1. Mix the egg whites with the tartar cream in a bowl and swerve and swirl using your mixer.
2. Whisk the cream with the vanilla extract in another bowl and mix thoroughly.
3. Combine and gently whisk the two mixtures.
4. Whisk the egg yolks very well in another bowl and then apply the combination of two egg whites.
5. Gently stir, put it into a container and leave it in the refrigerator for 3 hours until the ice cream is eaten.

6.

Chapter 12- Smoothie Recipes

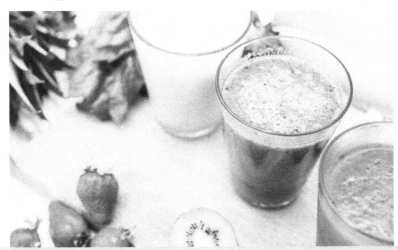

12.1 Minted Iced Berry Sparkler

Ready in about 30 minutes | Servings-2 | Difficulty-Easy

Ingredients

- One cup of mixed frozen berries
- One lime or lemon
- One cup of fresh mint
- Twenty drops liquid Stevia extract (Clear / Berry)
- One large bottle of water
- Ice

Instructions

1. Wash the mint.
2. Cut the lime into wedges that are thin.
3. Using your option of sparkling or still water to put mint, frozen berries, lemon wedges or lime and leftover ingredients into all in a jar.
4. Let yourself relax for 15 minutes or more. The longer you keep it, the taste gets bolder.
5. Serve.

12.2 Body Pumping Smoothie

Ready in about 10 minutes | Servings-2 | Difficulty-Easy

Ingredients

- One beetroot
- One Apple
- Three tablespoons of yogurt
- Handful of mint
- One thumb of a two-inch ginger
- Half teaspoon of black salt or rock salt
- One teaspoon of honey or sugar
- A quarter cup of water

Instructions

1. Clean and remove the beet peel.
2. Slice the medium-sized apple and remove the nuts.
3. Add all the ingredients into the blender.
4. Add ice, then proceed to mix into a paste that is smooth.
5. Add juice from the lemon.
6. Enjoy and serve.

12.3 Kiwi Dream Blender

Ready in about 10 minutes | Servings-2 | Difficulty-Easy

Ingredients

- A quarter average avocado
- One small wedge of Galia melon (or Honeydew, Cantaloupe)
- One scoop of vanilla whey protein powder (vanilla or plain)
- powdered gelatin
- Six drops liquid Stevia extract
- Ice as per the need
- A quarter cups of coconut milk (or coconut cream or full-fat cream)
- A quarter cup of kiwi berries or kiwi fruit
- One tablespoon of chia seeds (or psyllium)
- Half cups of water

Instructions

1. Strip and peel the avocado and put it in a blender.
2. Add the kiwi, melon and the remaining ingredients to the flesh.
3. Blend until completely smooth.
4. Serve.

12.4 Keto Smart Banana Blender

Ready in about 10 minutes | Servings-2 | Difficulty-Easy

Ingredients

- One cup of Spinach
- One cup of Banana
- Half cup of water and yogurt
- Two tablespoons of Pomegranate
- Two tablespoons of Almond meal/ Almonds
- One teaspoon of Cinnamon powder
- One teaspoon of Vanilla sugar or Honey or Sugar and vanilla extract
- Ice

Instructions

1. Clean the spinach and chop it coarsely.
2. Cut the Banana into medium-sized portions.
3. To make a half-cup of milk, blend two to three tablespoons of yogurt with water.
4. In a blender, mix all ingredients and process until smooth.
5. If the ideal thickness is met, add ice when blending.

6. Then serve.

12.5 Bright Morning Smoothie

Ready in about 15 minutes | Servings-2 | Difficulty-Easy

Ingredients

- Two cups of Washed Spinach
- Two Large Strawberries
- A quarter cup of Lemon Juice or Fresh Squeezed Orange Juice
- Two tablespoons of Chia Seeds or Powder
- One cup of Green Tea
- One cup of Ice
- Four tablespoons of sweetener of choice

Instructions

1. Place all of the ingredients in a mixer.
2. Blend it all until smooth.
3. Let it rest for about 5-10 minutes, then serve.

12.6 Keto Iced Strawberry and Greens

Ready in about 10 minutes | Servings-2 | Difficulty-Easy

Ingredients

- Half cup coconut water
- One cup of ice
- One cup of washed spinach
- Three large strawberries
- Sweetener to taste

Instructions

1. Blend all the ingredients together in a blender until smooth.
2. Let it rest for 5 minutes and then serve chilled.

12.7 Strawberry Lime Ginger Punch

Ready in about 10 minutes | Servings-2 | Difficulty-Easy

Ingredients

- Two cups of water
- Two tablespoons of raw apple cider vinegar
- Three packets of NuStevia or any other sweetener
- Juice of one lime
- Half teaspoon of ginger powder
- Five frozen strawberries

Instructions

1. Blend all the ingredients together in a blender until smooth.
2. Let it rest for 5 minutes and then serve chilled.

12.8 Mexican Comfort Cream

Ready in about 20 minutes | Servings-2 | Difficulty-Easy

Ingredients

- Two handfuls of almonds blanched
- One cup of almond milk (unsweetened)
- One large egg
- Two tablespoons of whole or ground chia seeds
- One tablespoon of lime zest
- One teaspoon of cinnamon powder or one whole cinnamon stick
- Three tablespoons of erythritol or another healthy low-carb sweetener
- Twenty drops of liquid Stevia extract (Clear / Cinnamon)
- Two cups of warm water

Instructions

1. Put in a bowl lime zest, the blanched almonds and cinnamon stick and cover with two teaspoons of hot water.
2. Let it rest for about eight hours or overnight.
3. Remove the lime zest and cinnamon stick after the almonds have been softened and put them in a shallow saucepan.
4. Mix almond milk. Purée until it's really smooth.
5. Steam the mixture and mix cinnamon and sweeteners before it begins to sizzle.
6. Whisk the egg when stirring constantly and pour it gently into the mixture.
7. Stir for a minute or two over the sun.
8. Remove from the heat and add in the seeds of chia.
9. To thicken the remainder.
10. Serve cold and pour in a bottle.

12.9 Strawberry Protein Smoothie

Ready in about 10 minutes | Servings-2 | Difficulty-Easy

Ingredients

- Half cup water
- One cup of ice
- One scoop of strawberry protein powder
- One egg
- Two tablespoons of cream
- Two strawberries

Instructions

1. Blend ice cubes and water together.
2. Apply the egg, powder and strawberries and start blending.
3. Pour in the cream.
4. Blend it again until smooth in a blender.
5. Serve and enjoy.

12.10 Low-Carb Caribbean Cream

Ready in about 2 hours and 10 minutes | Servings-1 | Difficulty-Moderate

Ingredients

- Half cup of unsweetened coconut milk
- A quarter cups of coconut water or water (iced)
- One shot of dark or white rum
- One slice of fresh pineapple
- Five drops of liquid Stevia extract

Instructions

1. In an ice cube tray, freeze the coconut water for 1-2 hours.
2. Blend coconut milk and pineapple until creamy.
3. Add the coconut water ice cubes and rum to the serving bottle.
4. Add the combined solution.
5. Use the pineapple to garnish.
6. Serve and enjoy.

Conclusion

The ketogenic diet comprises a low-carbohydrate, high-protein and high-fat diet with a lengthy history of use in the management of intractable childhood seizures. Amid the existence of growing quantities of modern antiepileptic medications and surgical therapies, this nutritional therapy has enjoyed increasing success in recent years.

The authors study the past of the ketogenic diet, its conventional initiation protocol, potential modes of operation, proof of success, and side effects. In particular, several of the fields of an ongoing study in this area are illustrated, as are potential paths and unresolved issues.

An efficient and reasonably healthy cure for intractable epilepsy is the ketogenic diet. However, considering its lengthy past, everything regarding the diet, including its modes of operation, the optimum protocol, and the complete extent of its applicability, remains unclear. Diet study offers fresh insight into the causes underlying epilepsy and seizures itself, as well as potential possible approaches.

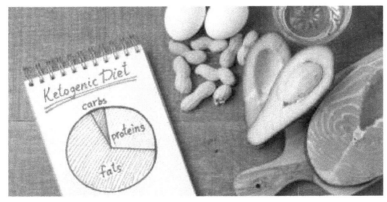

It would not be unreasonable to claim that when it comes to intermittent fasting, there is little to fear. While at first, you will feel starving, by triggering autophagy and losing more fat and ketones for food, your body will adapt.

A longer intermittent fast accompanied by shorter regular intermittent fasts is proposed by ketogenic diet researchers. In the days preceding and during the three-day fast, you will use a fasting regimen that involves fasting for up to three days, 3 to 4 times a year, with a shorter 10 to 18 hour fast.

If you are fasting for sixteen hours or three days to prevent symptoms of refeeding syndrome, checking your mineral levels is crucial.

To prevent unnecessary mineral depletion induced by ketogenic diets and fasting, supplementation of sodium from unprocessed potassium and salt, phosphate, and magnesium from mineral-rich foods or supplements could be essential.

 To put an end to it, it won't be wrong to say that the Ketogenic Diet is a miraculous diet as it focuses on healthy starvation and lets the body utilize the already stored fat and fastens the weight loss procedure as the intake of calories is less and the already stored fat is converted into energy by the body.

Keto Dessert & Chaffle Cookbook 2021 with Pictures

Quick and Easy, Sugar-Low Bombs, Chaffle and Cakes Recipes to Shed Weight, Boost Your Mood and Live Ketogenic lifestyle

By
Gianna Carter

Table of Contents

Introduction

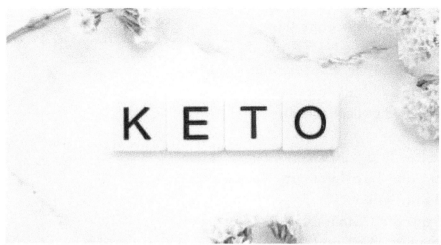

The ketogenic diet or Keto is a low-carbohydrate, mild protein, high-fat diet that will help you lose fat more efficiently. It has several advantages for weight reduction, wellbeing, and efficiency, so a rising number of healthcare professionals & practitioners recommend it.

Fat as a form of nutrition

For nutrition, the body uses three fuel sources: carbohydrates, fats and proteins. Carbohydrates convert into blood sugar or glucose in the bloodstream and are the primary fuel source for the body. If carbohydrates are not accessible, your body then depends on fat as an energy source. Protein is the primary building block of muscles and tissues. Protein could also be processed into glucose in a pinch and utilized for energy.

The keto diet encourages your body to utilize fat as the primary source of nutrition instead of carbohydrates, a ketosis mechanism. You consume too little carbs on the keto diet that the body cannot depend on glucose for nutrition. And your body turns to utilize fat for energy rather than carbs, as keto foods are filled with fat. A major part of the calories, almost 70 to 80% come from fat, consuming 15 to 20% of calories from protein and barely 5% calories from carbohydrates (that makes for about 20 to 30 grams of carbohydrates per day, depending on the weight and height of a person).

Meal options in regular diets

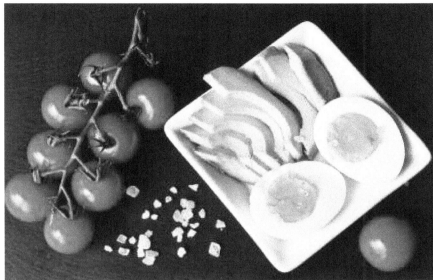

To conquer the weight reduction fight, it becomes tough to continue the dieting combat for a long period. Many people revert to the previous eating patterns after only a few weeks when confronted with the difficulty and limited food ranges of many diets, especially vegan, low-fat and low-calorie diets. For starters, the ketogenic diet is incredibly beneficial for weight reduction, but following specific food choices can be overwhelming. Only after three weeks can you begin noticing significant effects; however, the complications and inconvenience of transitioning to an effective ketogenic diet may deter you from keeping to the program long enough to reap the benefits.

Thankfully, to render your keto diet ever more efficient, successful and simple to use, you will build an array of foods, preparing strategies, tips and suggestions. One hidden tool can be used from the diet's outset, without much details of the keto diet, which is continued even after achieving the weight loss target.

That hidden preferred weapon is the "Fat Bomb."

The Fat Bomb

The fat bombs in the keto diet play a major role in motivation for the dieters. Indulging in a high fat dessert gives you a stress-free environment to continue your diet. These fat bombs provide the correct amounts of fat, carbohydrates, and protein resulting in weight reduction while supplying the user with sustained energy. They do this by supplementing your diet with chemicals that hold your body in a fat-burning state, even after you have had a fulfilling meal.

The Keto diet aims to rely on foods that are high in fat and low in carbs. By modifying what the body utilizes as food, it helps facilitate weight reduction. Carbohydrates, like those present in sugars and bread, are usually transformed into energy. If the body cannot have enough nutrients, the body begins to burn fat as a substitute for energy.

Your liver converts the fat into ketones, which are a form of acid. Getting a certain amount of ketones in your body will lead you to a biochemical condition known as ketosis. Your body can burn stored fat for fuel; thus, you will losing weight when you go through ketosis.

To reach a ketosis condition, it takes between one to ten days of consuming a low-carb, high-fat diet; to sustain the fat-burning cycle of ketosis, you have to continue consuming the keto diet. Eating fatty foods will help you more easily get into ketosis and sustain it for longer periods.

Fat bombs are 90% fat, making them the ideal keto addition for beginners and lifetime keto adherents. They hold you in a ketosis state and can provide health advantages unlike many other high protein foods; you can snack on fat bombs or have them as dinners or as have as a side dish too. They are simple to produce and are available in a range of varieties, from sweet to savory.

Can Fat Bombs Be Healthy?
Ketogenic fat bombs are fueled by two major ingredients: high-fat dairy and coconut oil. Both of these components have several powerful health advantages. Coconut produces a form of fat known as MCTs (medium-chain triglycerides), which gives the body additional ketones that can be readily consumed and used to sustain ketosis.

There are distinct health advantages of consuming high-fat dairy fat bombs. High-fat dairy products produce fatty acids known as CLA (conjugated linoleic acid), minerals and vitamins. Data indicates that CLA plays a significant role in the body's breakdown of fat and may lower cardiac attack and stroke risk.

Eating high-fat dairy meals prior to bedtime may help burn fat when still sleeping. Fat burned while you sleep the body with an energy that does not need to metabolize stress hormones or depend on sugar.

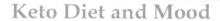

Keto Diet and Mood

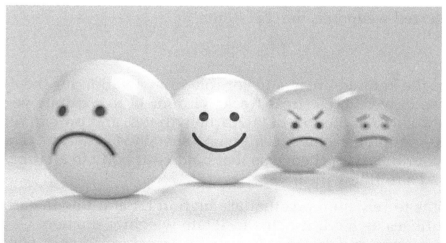

There are various comments from individuals on a keto diet that probably indicate the association between the keto diet and mood changes. Various hypotheses connect the keto diet to mood regulation, even if only partly.

The explanation of why the keto diet aids in accelerated weight reduction and reversal of multiple chronic weight-related problems lead people to come out of the despair of "I am not healthy." As a consequence of the results themselves, most people report a positive attitude by adopting a keto diet. But is that important? What makes a difference is that it has a positive and long-lasting effect. Some research also shows that a ketogenic diet may help combat depression since it provides anti-inflammatory benefits. Inflammations are associated with, at least certain, forms of depression. A few of the advantages are provided below that create the relationship between the keto diet and mood. A keto diet:

1. Helps regulate energy highs and lows.

Ketones offer an immediate energy supply for your brain since they are metabolized quicker than glucose. Ketones give a long-lasting, more accurate and reliable energy supply, and when your body understands it can access your fat reserves for food as well, the brain does not worry.

2. Neurogenesis improvement

Dietary consumption is a crucial element in assessing neurogenesis. A reduced degree of neurogenesis is correlated with multiple depressive illnesses. On the other side, a higher rate increases emotional endurance.

3. Reduces and Brings Down Inflammation

The Keto Diet provides healthy nutritional options, so you avoid consuming inflammatory and refined products. Consuming anti-inflammatory food can have a direct impact on the attitude. If you eat nutritious food high in protein, healthy fats and low-carb vegetables, it reduces inflammation.

4. Feeds the brain.

The good fat you consume on Keto fuels your brain and stabilizes your mood. As your brain is composed of 60% fat, it requires an excess of healthy fats to function properly.

So go ahead and try these easy to make lo carb hi fat desserts and lose weight deliciously!

Chapter 1- Low Carb Desserts

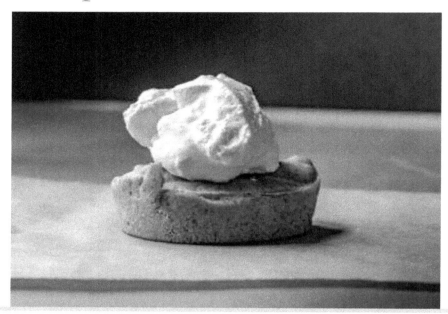

1. 10 Minutes Chocolate Mousse

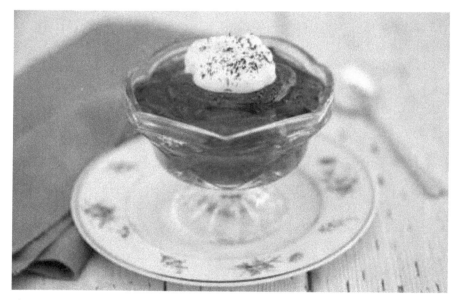

Prep. Time: 10 minutes

Servings: 4

The serving size is ½ cup

Nutrition as per serving:

218 kcal / 23g fat / 5g carbs / 2g fiber / 2g protein = 3g net carbs

Ingredients

- Powdered sweetener 1/4 cup
- Cocoa powder, unsweetened, sifted 1/4 cup

- Vanilla extract 1tsp.
- Heavy whipping cream 1 cup
- Kosher salt 1/4tsp.

Directions

With an electric beater, beat the cream to form stiff peaks. Put in the sweetener, cocoa powder, salt, vanilla and whisk till all ingredients are well combined.

2. The Best Keto Cheesecake

Prep. Time: 20 minutes

Cook Time: 50 minutes

Setting Time: 8 hours

Servings: 12

The serving size is 1 slice

Nutrition as per serving:

600kcal / 54g fat / 7g carbs / 2g fiber / 14g protein = 5 g net carbs

Ingredients

Layer of crust

- Powdered sweetener 1/4 cup
- Almond flour 1 1/2 cups
- Butter melted 6 tbsp.
- Cinnamon 1tsp.

Filling

- Cream cheese, full fat, room temperature (8 oz.)
- Powdered Sweetener 2 Cups
- Eggs at room temperature 5 Large
- Sour cream at room temperature 8 Oz.
- Vanilla extract 1 Tbsp.

Directions

1. Heat the oven to 325F.
2. Arrange the rack in the center of the oven. Mix dry ingredients for the crust in a medium mixing bowl. Mix in the butter. Transfer the crust mixture into a springform pan (10-inch x 4- inch), and using your fingers, press halfway up and around the sides. Then press the mixture with a flat bottom cup into the pan. Chill the crust for about 20 minutes.
3. Beat the cream cheese (at room temperature) in a large mixing container, with an electric beater or a
4. Hand mixer until fluffy and light.
5. If using a stand mixer, attach the paddle accessory.
6. Add in about 1/3rd of sweetener at a time and beat well.
7. Add in one egg at a time beating until well incorporated.

8. Lastly, add in the sour cream, vanilla and mix until just combined.
9. Pour this cheesecake mixture onto the crust and smooth out the top. Place in the heated oven and examine after 50 minutes. The center should not jiggle, and the top should not be glossy anymore.
10. Turn the oven off and open the door slightly, leaving the cheesecake inside for about 30 minutes.
11. Take out the cheesecake and run a knife between the pan and the cheesecake (this is to unstick the cake but don't remove the springform yet). Leave for 1 hour.
12. Chill for at least 8 hrs. loosely covered with plastic wrap.
13. Take off the sides of the springform pan, decorate & serve.

Note: all the ingredients to make the cheesecake should be at room temperature. Anything refrigerated must be left out for at least 4 hrs.

3. Butter Pralines

Prep. Time: 5 minutes

Cook Time: 11 minutes

Chilling Time: 1 hour

Servings: 10

The serving size is 2 Butter Pralines

Nutrition as per serving:

338kcal / 36g fat / 3g carbs / 2g fiber / 2g protein = 1g net carbs

Ingredients

- Salted butter 2 Sticks
- Heavy Cream 2/3 Cup
- Granular Sweetener 2/3 Cup
- Xanthan gum ½ tsp.
- Chopped pecans 2 Cups
- Sea salt

Directions

1. Line parchment paper on a cookie sheet with or apply a silicone baking mat on it.
2. In a saucepan, brown the butter on medium-high heat, stirring regularly, for just about 5 minutes.
3. Add in the sweetener, heavy cream and xanthan gum. Stir and take off the heat.
4. Add in the nuts and chill to firm up, occasionally stirring, for about 1 hour. The mixture will become very thick. Shape into ten cookie forms and place on the lined baking sheet, and sprinkle with the sea salt, if preferred. Let chill until hardened.
5. Keep in a sealed container, keep refrigerated until serving.

4. Homemade Healthy Twix Bars

Prep. Time: 5 minutes

Cook Time: 20 minutes

Servings: 18 Bars

The serving size is 1 Bar

Nutrition as per serving:

111kcal / 7g fat / 8g carbs / 5g fiber / 4g protein = 3g net carbs

Ingredients

For the cookie layer

- Coconut flour 3/4 cup
- Almond flour 1 cup
- Keto maple syrup 1/4 cup
- Sweetener, granulated 1/2 cup
- Flourless keto cookies 1/4 cup
- Almond milk 1/2 cup

For the gooey caramel

- Cashew butter (or any seed or nut butter) 1 cup
- Sticky sweetener of choice 1 cup
- Coconut oil 1 cup
- For the chocolate coating
- Chocolate chips 2 cups

Directions

1. Line parchment paper in a loaf pan or square pan and set aside.
2. In a big mixing bowl, put in almond flour, coconut flour, and then granulated. Combine very well. Mix in the keto syrup and stir to make it into a thick dough.
3. Add the crushed keto cookies and also add a tbsp. of milk to keep it a thick batter. If the batter stays too thick, keep adding milk by tablespoon. Once desired consistency is achieved, shift the batter to the prepared pan and smooth it out. Chill.
4. Combine the cashew butter, coconut oil and syrup on the stovetop or a microwave-safe dish and heat until mixed. Beat very well to make sure the coconut oil is completely mixed. Drizzle the caramel over the prepared cookie layer and shift to the freezer.
5. When the bars are hard, take out of the pan and slice into 18 bars. Once more, put it back in the freezer.
6. Liquefy the chocolate chips by heat. Using two forks, dip each Twix bar into the melted chocolate till evenly covered. Cover all the bars with chocolate. Chill until firm.

5. Best Chocolate Chip cookie

Prep. Time: 5 minutes

Cook Time: 20 minutes

Servings: 15 Cookies

The serving size is 1 Cookie

Nutrition as per serving:

98kcal / 6g fat / 12g carbs / 5g fiber / 5g protein = 7g net carbs

Ingredients

- Almond flour blanched 2 cups
- Baking powder 1 tsp
- Cornstarch 1/4 cup
- Coconut oil 2 tbsp.
- Sticky sweetener, keto-friendly 6 tbsp.
- Almond extract 1 tsp
- Coconut milk, unsweetened 1/4 cup
- Chocolate chips 1/2 cup

Directions

1. Heat oven up to 350F/175C. Line parchment paper on a large cookie tray and put it aside.
2. Place all the dry ingredients in a big mixing bowl, and combine well.
3. Melt the keto-friendly-sticky sweetener, almond extract and coconut oil in a microwave-safe proof or stovetop. Then mix it into the dry mixture, adding milk to combine very well. Stir through your chocolate chips.
4. Form small balls with slightly wet hands from the cookie dough. Set the balls up on the lined cookie tray. Then form them into cookies by pressing them with a fork. Bake for 12 to 15 minutes till they brown.
5. Take out from the oven, allowing to cool on the tray completely.

6. White Chocolate Dairy Free Peanut Butter Cups

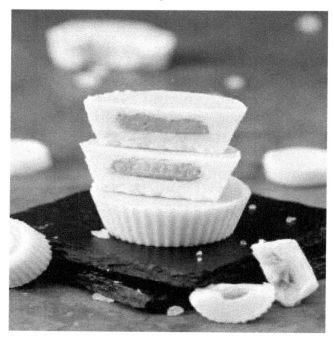

Prep. Time: 5 minutes

Cook Time: 5 minutes

Servings: 40

The serving size is 1 cup

Nutrition as per serving:

117kcal / 6g fat / 14g carbs / 10g fiber / 3g protein = 4g net carbs

Ingredients

- White Chocolate Bar, Sugar-free, coarsely chopped 4 cups
- Peanut butter, smooth (or sunflower seed butter) 1 cup
- Coconut flour 2 tbsp.
- Unsweetened coconut milk 2 tbsp.+ more if needed

Directions

1. Line muffin liners in a standard muffin tin of 12 cups or mini muffin tin of 20 cups and put aside.
2. Removing ½ a cup of your white chocolate, melt the remaining 3 1/2 cups on the stovetop or in a microwave-safe dish, till silky and smooth. Quickly, pour the melted white chocolate equally amongst the prepared muffin cups, scrape down the sides to remove all. Once done, chill
3. Meanwhile, start making the peanut butter filling. Mix the flour and peanut butter well. Adding a tsp. of milk at a time brings to the desired texture.
4. Take the hardened white chocolate cups, then equally pour the peanut butter filling among all of them. After all, is used up, take white chocolate that was kept aside and melt them. Then pour it on each of the cups to cover fully. Chill until firm.

7. Chocolate Crunch Bars

Prep. Time: 5 minutes

Cook Time: 5 minutes

Servings: 20 servings

The serving size is 1 Bar

Nutrition as per serving:

155kcal / 12g fat / 4g carbs / 2g fiber / 7g protein = 2g net carbs

Ingredients

- Chocolate chips (stevia sweetened), 1 1/2 cups
- Almond butter (or any seed or nut butter) 1 cup
- Sticky sweetener (swerve sweetened or monk fruit syrup) 1/2 cup
- Coconut oil 1/4 cup
- Seeds and nuts (like almonds, pepitas, cashews, etc.) 3 cups

Directions

1. Line parchment paper on a baking dish of 8 x 8-inch and put it aside.
2. Combine the keto-friendly chocolate chips, coconut oil, almond butter and sticky sweetener and melt on a stovetop or a microwave-safe dish until combined.

3. Include nuts and seeds and combine until fully mixed. Pour this mixture into the parchment-lined baking dish smoothing it out with a spatula. Chill until firm.

Notes

Keep refrigerated

8. Easy Peanut Butter Cups

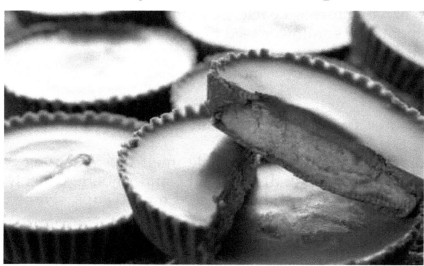

Prep. Time: 10minutes

Cook Time: 5minutes

Servings: 12

The serving size is 1 piece

Nutrition as per serving:

187kcal / 18g fat / 14g carbs / 11g fiber / 3g protein = 3g net carbs

Ingredients

Chocolate layers

- Dark chocolate(not bakers chocolate), Sugar-free, 10 oz. Divided
- Coconut oil 5 tbsp. (divided)
- Vanilla extracts 1/2 tsp. (divided) optional

Peanut butter layer

- Creamy Peanut butter 3 1/2 tbsp.
- Coconut oil 2 tsp.
- Powdered Erythritol (or to taste) 4 tsp.
- Peanut flour 1 1/2 tsp.
- Vanilla extracts 1/8 tsp. Optional
- Sea salt 1 pinch (or to taste) optional

Directions

1. Line parchment liners in a muffin pan

2. Prepare the chocolate layer on the stove, place a double boiler and heat half of the coconut oil and half of the chocolate, stirring regularly, until melted. (Alternatively use a microwave, heat for 20 seconds, stirring at intervals.). Add in half of the vanilla.
3. Fill each lined muffin cup with about 2 tsp. Of chocolate in each. Chill for around 10 minutes till the tops are firm.
4. Prepare the peanut butter filling: in a microwave or a double boiler, heat the coconut oil and peanut butter (similar to step 2). Mix in the peanut flour, powdered sweetener, sea salt and vanilla until smooth. Adjust salt and sweetener to taste if preferred.
5. Pour a tsp. Of the prepared peanut mixture into each cup with the chocolate layer. You don't want it to reach the edges. Chill for 10 minutes more till the tops are firm.
6. Now, prepare a chocolate layer for the top. Heat the leftover coconut oil and chocolate in a microwave or the double boiler (similar to step 2). Add in the vanilla.
7. Pour about 2 tsp of melted chocolate into each cup. It should cover the empty part and the peanut butter circles completely.
8. Again chill for at least 20 to 30 minutes, until completely solid. Keep in the refrigerator.

9. No-Bake Chocolate Coconut Bars

Prep. Time: 1 minute

Cook Time: 5 minutes

Servings: 12 bars

The serving size is 1 bar

Nutrition as per serving:

169 kcal / 17g fat / 5g carbs / 4g fiber / 2g protein = 1g net carbs

Ingredients

- Keto maple syrup 1/4 cup
- Coconut unsweetened, shredded 3 cups
- Coconut oil, melted 1 cup
- Lily's chocolate chips 1-2 cups

Directions

1. Line parchment paper in a large loaf pan or square pan and put aside.
2. Add all the ingredients to a large bowl and combine very well. Shift mixture to the prepared pan. Wet your hands lightly and press them into place. Chill for 30 minutes until firm. Cut into 12 bars.
3. Melt the sugar-free chocolate chips, and using two forks, dip each chilled bar into the melted chocolate and coat evenly. Evenly coat all the bars in the same way. Chill until chocolate solidifies.
4. Keep the Bars in a sealed container at room temperature. If you refrigerated or freeze them, thaw them completely before enjoying them.

10. Chocolate Peanut Butter Hearts

Prep. Time: 5 minutes

Cook Time: 5 minutes

Servings: 20 Hearts

The serving size is 1 Heart

Nutrition as per serving:

95kcal / 6g fat / 7g carbs / 5g fiber / 5g protein = 2g net carbs

Ingredients

- Smooth peanut butter 2 cups
- Sticky sweetener 3/4 cup
- Coconut flour 1 cup
- Chocolate chips of choice 1-2 cups

Directions

1. Line parchment paper on a large tray and put it aside.
2. Combine the keto-friendly sticky sweetener and peanut butter and melt on a stovetop or microwave-safe bowl until combined.
3. Include coconut flour and combine well. If the mixture is too thin, include more coconut flour. Leave for around 10 minutes to thicken.
4. Shape the peanut butter mixture into 18 to 20 small balls. Press each ball in. Then, using a heart-molded cookie cutter, shape the balls into hearts removing excess peanut butter mixture from the sides. Assemble the hearts on the lined tray and chill.
5. Melt the keto-friendly chocolate chips. With two forks, coat the chocolate by dipping each heart into it. Repeat with all hearts. When done, chill until firm.

Notes

Keep in a sealed jar at room temperature for up to 2 weeks, or refrigerate for up to 2 months.

11. Magic Cookies

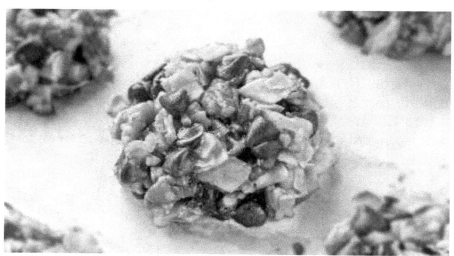

Prep. Time: 10 minutes

Cook Time: 15 minutes

Servings: 15 cookies

The serving size is 1 cookie

Nutrition as per serving:

130kcal / 13g fat / 2g carbs / 1g fiber / 2g protein = 1g net carbs

Ingredients

- Butter softened 3 tbsp.
- Coconut oil 1/4 cup
- Granulated swerve sweetener 3 tbsp.
- Dark chocolate chips, sugar-free (like lily's) 1 cup
- Egg yolks 4 large
- Coconut flakes 1 cup
- Kosher salt 1/2 tsp.
- Walnuts roughly chopped 3/4 cup.

Directions

1. Heat oven up to 350° and line a parchment paper on a baking sheet. In a large mixing bowl, whisk together butter, coconut oil, sweetener, egg yolks and salt; stir in walnuts, coconut, and chocolate chips.
2. Drop spoonfuls of batter onto the prepared baking sheet. Place in the oven and bake for 15 mins until golden,

12. No-Bake Coconut Crack Bars

Prep. Time: 2 minutes

Cook Time: 3 minutes

Servings: 20

The serving size is 1 square

Nutrition as per serving:

108kcal / 11g fat / 2g carbs / 2g fiber /2g protein = 0g net carbs

Ingredients

- Coconut flakes unsweetened & Shredded 3 cups
- Coconut oil, melted 1 cup
- Maple syrup, monk fruit sweetened 1/4 cup (or any liquid sweetener of preference)

Directions

1. Line parchment paper on an 8 x 10-inch pan or an 8 x 8-inch pan and put aside. Or use a loaf pan.

2. Combine unsweetened shredded coconut, melted coconut oil, maple syrup (monk fruit sweetened) in a big mixing bowl and mix till you get a thick batter. If you find it crumbling, add a tsp. of water or a bit of extra syrup.
3. Transfer the coconut mixture to the lined pan. Press firmly with slightly wet hands into place. Chill until firmed. Cut into bars & enjoy!

13. Candied Pecans

Prep. Time: 5 minutes

Cook Time: 1 minute

Servings: 16 Servings

The serving size is 1 Serving

Nutrition as per serving:

139kcal / 15g fat / 3g carbs / 2g fiber / 2g protein = 1g net carbs

Ingredients

- Granulated sweetener divided 1 1/2 cups
- Vanilla extract 1 tsp
- Water 1/4 cup
- Cinnamon 1 tbsp.
- Raw pecans 3 cups

Directions

1. Over medium flame, heat a skillet or large pan.
2. Add 1 cup of the granulated sweetener, vanilla extract and water, and stir until fully mixed. Let it heat up, stirring in between.
3. Once the sweetener is fully melted, include your pecans. Stir around the pecans ensuring every nut is equally coated in the liquid mixture. Keep occasionally stirring till the sweetener starts to set on the pecans. Take off from the heat. Leave for 2 to 3 minutes.
4. Brea apart the pecans with a wooden spoon before they set together.
5. When cooled, mix with the granulated sweetener that was reserved earlier and cinnamon. Store in a sealed container.

14. Sugar-Free Flourless Cookies

Prep. Time: 2 minutes

Cook Time: 10 minutes

Servings: 14 cookies

The serving size is 1 Cookie

Nutrition as per serving:

101kcal / 9g fat / 3g carbs / 1g fiber / 5g protein = 3g net carbs

Ingredients

For the original style:

- Almond butter 1 cup
- Egg 1 large
- Granulated sweetener, stevia blend monk fruit, 3 /4 cup

For the egg-free style:

- Almond butter smooth 1 cup
- Chia seeds, ground 3-4 tbsp.
- Granulated sweetener, stevia blend monk fruit 3/4 cup

Directions

1. Heat the oven up to 350 degrees. Place parchment paper on a cookie sheet or a baking tray.
2. In a big mixing bowl, add all the ingredients and blend until well combined. When using the egg-free recipe, begin with 3 tbsps. of grounded chia seeds. Add an extra tbsp. if the mixture is still too thin.
3. Using your hands or a cookie scoop, shape small balls and place them 3 to 4 inches apart on the baking tray. Make into cookie shape by pressing down with a fork. Bake until cookies are beginning to get a golden brown color but still soft, or for 8 to 10 minutes. Take out from the oven, allowing to cool until firm but soft and chewy.

15. Salted Caramel Fudge

Prep. Time: 5 minutes

Cook Time: 5 minutes

Servings: 24 servings

The serving size is 1 fudge cup

Nutrition as per serving:

148kcal / 15g fat / 4g carbs / 2g fiber / 4g protein = 2g net carbs

Ingredients

- Cashew butter 2 cups
- Keto maple syrup 1/4 cup
- Coconut oil 1/2 cup

Directions

1. Line muffin liners in a mini muffin tin of 24-count and put aside.
2. Combine all the ingredients on a stovetop or in a microwave-safe dish and heat till melted.
3. Take off from heat and beat very well till a glossy, smooth texture remains.

4. Split the fudge mixture equally in the lined muffin tin. Chill for about 30 minutes, till firm.

16. Healthy Kit Kat Bars

Prep. Time: 5 minutes

Cook Time: 5 minutes

Servings: 20 Bars

The serving size is 1 Bar

Nutrition as per serving:

149kcal / 12g fat / 4g carbs / 2g fiber / 7g protein = 2g net carbs

Ingredients

- Keto granola 2 cups
- Almond butter (or any seed or nut butter) 1 cup
- Mixed seeds 1/2 cup
- Coconut oil 1/4 cup
- Mixed nuts 1/2 cup
- Dark chocolate chips, 1 1/2 cups
- Sticky sweetener 1/2 cup

Directions

1. Mix the mixed nuts, keto granola, and seeds in a big bowl. Put aside.
2. Melt the keto chocolate chips on the stovetop or in a microwave-safe dish. Include almond butter, coconut oil, and sticky sweetener. Heat until well combined.
3. Add the melted chocolate mixture onto the dry and combine until fully unified.
4. Shift the kit kat mixture to a pan of 10 x 10-inch lined with parchment. With a spatula, smooth out to a uniform layer. Chill for about 30 minutes, then slice into bars.

Notes: keep refrigerated

17. Healthy No-Bake Keto Cookie Bars

Prep. Time: 5 minutes

Cook Time: 25 minutes

Servings: 12 servings

The serving size is 1 Bar

Nutrition as per serving:

149kcal / 5g fat / 10g carbs / 6g fiber / 10g protein = 4g net carbs

Ingredients

For the cookie

- Almond flour blanched 1 1/2 cups
- Coconut flour 1/4 cup

- Cinnamon, a pinch
- Protein powder, vanilla flavor (optional) 2 scoops
- Granulated sweetener (like
- Sticky sweetener, keto-friendly, 1/2 cup
- Monk fruit sweetener) 2 tbsp.
- Vanilla extract 1/2 tsp
- Cashew butter (or any nut butter) 1/2 cup
- Sticky sweetener, keto-friendly, 1/2 cup
- Almond milk 1 tbsp.

For the protein icing

- Protein powder,
- Vanilla flavor 3 scoops
- Granulated sweetener, keto-friendly 1-2 tbsp. + for sprinkling 1/2 tsp
- Almond milk, (for batter) 1 tbsp.

For the coconut butter icing

- Coconut butter melted 4-6 tbsp.
- Sticky sweetener, 2 tbsp.
- Almond milk 1 tbsp.

Directions

1. Preparing sugar cookie base
2. Place tin foil in a baking pan of 8 x 8 inches and put aside.
3. Mix the protein powder, flours, granulated sweetener and cinnamon in a big mixing bowl, and put aside.
4. Melt the sticky sweetener with cashew butter on a stovetop or a microwave-proof bowl. Stir in the vanilla extract and add to the dry mixture. Beat superbly until fully combined. If the batter formed is too thick, add a tablespoon of almond milk with a tablespoon and mix well until desired consistency.
5. Pour the batter into the lined baking sheet and press tightly in place. Scatter the ½ teaspoon of keto-friendly granulated sweetener and chill for about 15 minutes until they are firm. Then add an icing of choice and chill for 30 minutes more to settle the icing before slicing.
6. Preparing the icing(s)
7. Mix all ingredients of the icings (separately) and, using almond milk, thin down the mixture till a very thick icing is formed.

18. Keto Chocolate Bark with Almonds and Bacon

Prep. Time: 30 minutes

Servings: 8 servings

The serving size is 1/8 of the recipe

Nutrition as per serving:

157kcal /12.8g fat / 4g protein / 7.5g fiber / 12.7g carbs = 5.2g net carbs

Ingredients

- Sugar-free Chocolate Chips 1 bag (9 oz.)
- Chopped Almonds 1/2 cup
- Bacon cooked & crumbled2 slices

Directions

1. In a microwave-safe bowl, melt the chocolate chips on high in 30 seconds intervals, stirring every time until all chocolate is melted.
2. Include the chopped almonds into the melted chocolate and mix.
3. Line a baking sheet with parchment and pour the chocolate mixture on it in a thin layer of about 1/2 inch.
4. Immediately top the chocolate with the crumbled bacon and press in with a flat spoon.
5. Chill for around 20 minutes or till the chocolate has solidified. Peel the parchment away from the hardened chocolate and crack it into eight pieces. Keep refrigerated.

Chapter 2- Chaffles

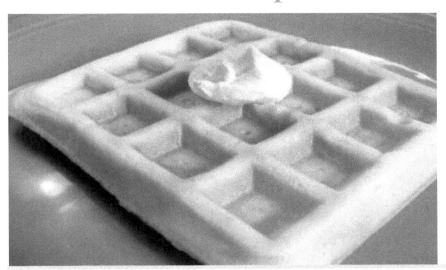

1. Basic chaffle recipe

Prep. Time: 5 minutes

Cook Time: 5 minutes

Servings: 1 chaffle

The serving size is 1 chaffle

Nutrition as per serving:

291kcal / 23g fat / 1g carbs / 0g fiber / 20g protein = 1g net carbs

Ingredients

• Sharp cheddar cheese shredded 1/2 cup
• Eggs 1

Directions

1. Whisk the egg.
2. In the waffle maker, assemble 1/4 cup of shredded cheese.
3. Top the cheese with beaten egg.
4. Top with the remainder 1/4 cup of cheese.
5. Cook till it's golden and crispy. It will get crispier as it cools.

2. Keto Oreo Chaffles

Prep. Time: 15 minutes

Cook Time: 8 minutes

Servings: 2 full-size chaffles or 4 mini chaffles

The serving size is 2 chaffles

Nutrition as per serving:

381kcal / 14.6g fat / 14g carbs / 5g fiber / 17g protein = 9g net carbs

Ingredients

- Sugar-Free Chocolate Chips 1/2 cup
- Butter 1/2 cup
- Eggs 3
- Truvia 1/4 cup
- Vanilla extract 1tsp.
- For Cream Cheese Frosting
- Butter, room temperature 4 oz.
- Cream Cheese, room temperature 4 oz.
- Powdered Swerve 1/2 cup
- Heavy Whipping Cream 1/4 cup
- Vanilla extract 1tsp.

Directions

1. Melt the butter and chocolate for around 1 minute in a microwave-proof dish. Stir well. You really ought to use the warmth within the chocolate and butter to melt most of the clumps. You have overheated the chocolate; when you microwave, and all is melted, it means you have overheated the chocolate. So grab yourself a spoon and begin stirring. If required, add 10 seconds, but stir just before you plan to do so.
2. Put the eggs, vanilla and sweetener, in a bowl and whisk until fluffy and light.
3. In a steady stream, add the melted chocolate into the egg mix and whisk again until well-combined.
4. In a Waffle Maker, pour around 1/4 of the mixture and cook for 7 to-8 minutes until it's crispy.
5. Prepare the frosting as they are cooking.
6. Put all the frosting ingredients into a food processor bowl and mix until fluffy and smooth. To achieve the right consistency, include a little extra cream.
7. To create your Oreo Chaffle, spread or pipe the frosting evenly in between the two chaffles.
8. The waffle machine, do not overfill it! It will create a giant mess and ruin the batter and the maker, utilizing no more than 1/4 cup of the batter.
9. Leave the waffles to cool down a bit before frosting. It is going to help them to remain crisp.
10. To make the frosting, use room-temp butter and cream cheese.

3. Glazed Donut Chaffle

Prep. Time: 10 mins

Cook Time: 5 mins

Servings: 3 chaffles

The serving size is 1 chaffle

Nutrition as per serving:

312kcal / 15g fat / 6g carbs / 1g fiber / 9g protein = 5g net carbs

Ingredients

For the chaffles

- Mozzarella cheese shredded ½ cup
- Whey protein isolates Unflavored 2 tbsp.
- Cream Cheese 1 oz.
- Swerve confectioners (Sugar substitute) 2 tbsp.
- Vanilla extract ½tsp.
- Egg 1
- Baking powder ½tsp.

For the glaze topping:

- Heavy whipping cream2 tbsp.
- Swerve confectioners (sugar substitute) 3-4 tbsp.
- Vanilla extract ½tsp.

Directions

1. Turn on the waffle maker.
2. In a microwave-proof bowl, combine the cream cheese and mozzarella cheese. Microwave at 30-second breaks until it is all melted and stir to combine completely.
3. Include the whey protein, baking powder, 2 tbsp. Keto sweetener to the melted cheese, and work with your hands to knead until well combined.
4. Put the dough in a mixing bowl, and whisk in the vanilla and egg into it to form a smooth batter.
5. Put 1/3 of the mixture into the waffle machine, and let it cook for 3 to 5 minutes.
6. Repeat the above step 5 to make a total of three chaffles.
7. Whisk the glaze topping ingredients together and drizzle on top of the chaffles generously before serving.

4. Keto Pumpkin Chaffles

Prep. Time: 2 mins

Cook Time: 5 mins

Servings: 2 chaffles

The serving size is 2 chaffles

Nutrition as per serving: (without toppings)

250kcal / 15g fat / 5g carbs / 1g fiber / 23g protein = 4g net carbs

Ingredients

- Mozzarella cheese, shredded ½ cup
- Egg, beaten 1 whole
- Pumpkin purée 1 ½ tbsp.

- Swerve confectioners ½tsp.
- Vanilla extract ½tsp.
- Pumpkin pie spice ¼tsp.
- Pure maple extract ⅛tsp.
- For topping- optional
- roasted pecans, cinnamon, whip cream and sugar-free maple syrup

Directions

1. Switch on the Waffle Maker and begin preparing the mixture.
2. Add all the given ingredients to a bowl, except for the mozzarella cheese, and whisk. Include the cheese and combine until well mixed.
3. Grease the waffle plates and put half the mixture into the middle of the plate. Cover the lid for 4- to 6 minutes, based on how crispy Chaffles you like.
4. Take it out and cook the second one. Serve with all or some mix of toppings, like sugar-free maple syrup, butter, roasted pecans, and a dollop of whipping cream or ground cinnamon dust.

5. Cream Cheese Chaffle with Lemon Curd

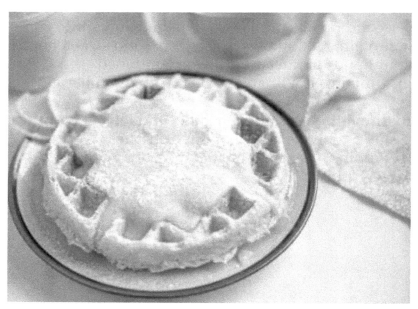

Prep. Time: 5 minutes

Cook Time: 4 minutes

Additional Time: 40 minute

Servings: 2-3 serving

The serving size is 1 chaffle

Nutrition as per serving:

302 kcals / 24g fat / 6g carbs / 1g fiber / 15g protein = 5g net carbs

Ingredients

- One batch keto lemon curd (recipe here)

- Eggs 3 large
- Cream cheese softened 4 oz.
- Lakanto monkfruit (or any low carb sweetener) 1 tbsp.
- Vanilla extract 1tsp.
- Mozzarella cheese shredded 3/4 cup
- Coconut flour 3 tbsp.
- Baking powder 1tsp.
- Salt 1/3tsp.
- Homemade keto whipped cream (optional) (recipe here)

Directions

1. Prepare lemon curd according to Directions and let cool in the refrigerator.
2. Turn on the waffle maker and grease it with oil.
3. Take a small bowl, put coconut flour, salt and baking powder. Combine and put aside.
4. Take a large bowl, put cream cheese, eggs, vanilla and sweetener. With an electric beater, beat until foamy. You may see chunks of cream cheese, and that is okay.
5. Include mozzarella cheese into the egg mixture and keep beating.
6. Pour the dry ingredients into the egg mixture and keep mixing until well blended.
7. Put batter into the preheated waffle machine and cook.
8. Take off from waffle machine; spread cooled lemon curd, top with keto whipped cream and enjoy.

6. Strawberries & Cream Keto Chaffles

Prep. Time: 25 minutes

Cook Time: 10 minutes

Servings: 8 chaffles

The serving size is 1 chaffle

Nutrition as per serving:

328cals / 12g fat / 8g carbs / 4g fiber / 6g protein = 4g net carbs

Ingredients

- Cream cheese 3 oz.
- Mozzarella cheese, shredded 2 cups
- Eggs, beaten 2
- Almond flour 1/2 cup
- Swerve confectioner sweetener 3 tbsp. + 1 tbsp.
- Baking powder 2tsps
- Strawberries 8
- Whipped cream 1 cup (canister - 2 tbsp. Per waffle)

Directions

1. In a microwavable dish, add the mozzarella and cream cheese, cook for 1 minute, mixing well. If the cheese is all melted, then go to the next step. Else cook for another 30 seconds stirring well.

2. Take another bowl, whisk eggs, including the almond flour, 3 tbsp. of keto sweetener, and baking powder.
3. Include the melted cheese mixture into the egg and almond flour mixture and combine well. Carefully add in 2 strawberries coarsely chopped. Chill for 20 minutes.
4. Meanwhile, slice the unused strawberries and mix with 1 tbsp. of Swerve. Chill.
5. Take out the batter from the refrigerator after 20 minutes. Heat the waffle iron and grease it.
6. Put 1/4 cup of the batter in the mid of the heated waffle iron. Ensuring the waffles are small makes it easier to remove from the waffle maker.
7. Transfer to a plate when cooked and cool before adding whipped cream and topping with strawberries.

This recipe gave me eight small waffles.

7. Keto Peanut Butter Cup Chaffle

Prep. Time: 2 minutes

Cook Time: 5 minutes

Servings: 2 Chaffles

The serving size is 1 chaffle + filling

Nutrition as per serving:

264kcal / 21.6g fat / 7.2g carbs / 2g fiber / 9.45g protein = 4.2g net carbs

Ingredients

For the Chaffle

- Heavy Cream 1 tbsp.
- Vanilla Extract 1/2 tsp
- Egg 1
- Cake Batter Flavor 1/2 tsp
- Unsweetened Cocoa 1 tbsp.
- Coconut Flour 1 tsp
- Lakanto Powdered Sweetener 1 tbsp.
- Baking Powder 1/4 tsp

For Peanut Butter Filling

- Heavy Cream 2 tbsp.
- All-natural Peanut Butter 3 tbsp.
- Lakanto Powdered Sweetener 2 tsp

Directions

1. Preheat a waffle maker.
2. Combine all the chaffle ingredients in a small mixing bowl.
3. Put half of the chaffle batter into the middle of the waffle machine and cook for 3 to 5 minutes.

4. Cautiously remove and duplicate for the second chaffle. Leave chaffles for a couple of minutes to let them crisp up.
5. Prepare the peanut butter filling by blending all the ingredients together and layer between chaffles.

8. Vanilla Chocolate Chip

Prep. Time: 1 minute

Cook Time: 4 minutes

Servings: 1 serving

The serving size is 1 large or 2 mini chaffle

Nutrition as per serving:

297.6 kcal. / 20.1g fat / 5.2g carbs / 1.5g fiber / 22.2g protein = 3.9g net carbs

Ingredients

- Mozzarella shredded 1/2 cup
- Eggs 1 medium
- Granulated sweetener keto 1 tbsp.
- Vanilla extract 1 tsp
- Almond meal or flour 2 tbsp.
- Chocolate chips, sugar-free 1 tbsp.

Directions

1. Mix all the ingredients in a large bowl.
2. Turn on the waffle maker. When it is heated, grease with olive oil and put half the mixture into the waffle machine. Cook for 2 to 4 minutes, then take out and repeat. It will make 2 small-chaffles per recipe.
3. Enjoy with your favorite toppings.

9. Chaffle Churro

Prep. Time: 10 minutes

Cook Time: 6-10 minutes

Servings: 2

The serving size is 4 churros

Nutrition as per serving:

189 kcals / 14.3g fat / 5.g carbs / 1g fiber / 10g protein = 4g net carbs

Ingredients

- Egg 1
- Almond flour 1 Tbsp.
- Vanilla extract ½ tsp.
- Cinnamon divided 1 tsp.
- Baking powder ¼ tsp.

- Shredded mozzarella ½ cup.
- Swerve confectioners (or any sugar substitute) 1 Tbsp.
- Swerve brown sugar (keto-friendly sugar substitute) 1 Tbsp.
- Butter melted 1 Tbsp.

Directions

1. Heat the waffle iron.
2. Combine the almond flour, egg, vanilla extract, baking powder, ½ tsp of cinnamon, swerve confectioners' sugar and shredded mozzarella in a bowl, and stir to combine well.
3. Spread half of the batter equally onto the waffle iron, and let it cook for 3 to 5 minutes. Cooking for more time will give a crispier chaffle.
4. Take out the cooked chaffle and pour the remaining batter onto it. Close the lid and cook for about 3 to 5 minutes.
5. Make both the chaffles into strips.
6. Put the cut strips in a bowl and drizzle on melted butter generously.
7. In another bowl, stir together the keto brown sugar and the leftover ½ tsp of cinnamon until well-combined.
8. Toss the churro chaffle strips in the sugar-cinnamon mixture in the bowl to coat them evenly.

10. Keto Cauliflower Chaffles Recipe

Prep. Time: 5 minutes

Cook Time: 4 minutes

Servings: 2 chaffles

The serving size is 2 chaffles

Nutrition as per serving:

246kcal / 16g fat / 7g carbs / 2g fiber / 20g protein = 5g net carbs

Ingredients

- Riced cauliflower 1 cup
- Garlic powder 1/4tsp.
- Ground black pepper 1/4tsp.
- Italian seasoning 1/2tsp.
- Kosher salt 1/4tsp.
- Mozzarella cheese shredded 1/2 cup
- Eggs 1
- Parmesan cheese shredded 1/2 cup

Directions

1. In a blender, add all the ingredients and blend well. Turn the waffle maker on.
2. Put 1/8 cup of parmesan cheese onto the waffle machine. Ensure to cover up the bottom of the waffle machine entirely.

3. Cover the cheese with the cauliflower batter, then sprinkle another layer of parmesan cheese on the cauliflower mixture. Cover and cook.
4. Cook for 4 to 5 minutes, or till crispy.
5. Will make 2 regular-size chaffles or 4 mini chaffles.
6. It freezes well. Prepare a big lot and freeze for the future.

11. Zucchini Chaffles

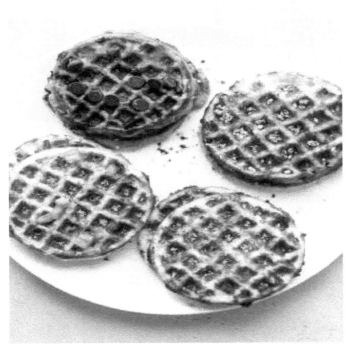

Prep. Time: 10 minutes

Cook Time: 5 minutes

Servings: 2 chaffles

The serving size is 1 chaffle

Nutrition as per serving:

194kcal / 13g fat / 4g carbs / 1g fiber / 16g protein = 3g net carbs

Ingredients

- Zucchini, grated 1 cup
- Eggs, beaten 1
- Parmesan cheese shredded 1/2 cup
- Mozzarella cheese shredded 1/4 cup
- Dried basil, 1tsp. Or fresh basil, chopped 1/4 cup
- Kosher Salt, divided 3/4tsp.
- Ground Black Pepper 1/2tsp.

Directions

1. Put the shredded zucchini in a bowl and Sprinkle salt, about 1/4tsp on it and leave it aside to gather other ingredients. Moments before using put the zucchini in a paper towel, wrap and press to wring out all the extra water.
2. Take a bowl and whisk in the egg. Include the mozzarella, grated zucchini, basil, and pepper 1/2tsp of salt.
3. Cover the waffle maker base with a layer of 1 to 2 tbsp. of the shredded parmesan.
4. Then spread 1/4 of the zucchini batter. Spread another layer of 1 to 2 tbsp. of shredded parmesan and shut the lid.
5. Let it cook for 4 to 8 minutes. It depends on the dimensions of your waffle machine. Normally, once the chaffle is not emitting vapors of steam, it is nearly done. For the greatest results, let it cook until good and browned.
6. Take out and duplicate for the next waffle.

Will make 4 small chaffles or 2 full-size chaffles in a Mini waffle maker.

12. Keto Pizza Chaffle

Prep. Time: 10 minutes

Cook Time: 30 minutes

Servings: 2 servings

The serving size is 1 chaffle

Nutrition as per serving:

76 kcal / 4.3g fat / 4.1g carbs / 1.2g fiber / 5.5g protein = 3.2g net carbs

Ingredients

- Egg 1
- Mozzarella cheese shredded 1/2 cup
- Italian seasoning a pinch
- Pizza sauce No sugar added 1 tbsp.
- Toppings – pepperoni, shredded cheese (or any other toppings)

Directions

- Heat the waffle maker.
- Whisk the egg, and Italian seasonings in a small mixing bowl, together.
- Stir in the cheese, leaving a few tsps. for layering.
- Layer a tsp of grated cheese onto the preheated waffle machine and allow it to cook for about 30 seconds.
- It will make a crispier crust.
- Pour half the pizza mixture into the waffle maker and allow to cook for around 4 minutes till it's slightly crispy and golden brown!
- Take out the waffle and make the second chaffle with the remaining mixture.
- Spread the pizza sauce, pepperoni and shredded cheese. Place in Microwave and heat on high for around 20 seconds and done! On the spot Chaffle PIZZA!

13. Crispy Taco Chaffle Shells

Prep. Time: 5 minutes

Cook Time: 8 minutes

Servings: 2 chaffles

The serving size is 1 chaffle

Nutrition as per serving:

258kcal / 19g fat / 4g carbs / 2g fiber / 18g protein = 2g net carbs

Ingredients

- Egg white 1
- Monterey jack cheese shredded 1/4 cup
- Sharp cheddar cheese shredded 1/4 cup
- Water 3/4 tsp
- Coconut flour 1 tsp
- Baking powder 1/4 tsp
- Chili powder 1/8 tsp
- Salt a pinch

Directions

1. Turn on the Waffle iron and lightly grease it with oil when it is hot.
2. In a mixing bowl, mix all of the above ingredients and blend to combine.
3. Pour half of the mixture onto the waffle iron and shut the lid. Cook for 4 minutes without lifting the lid. The chaffle will not set in less than 4 minutes.
4. Take out the cooked taco chaffle and put it aside. Do the same process with the remaining chaffle batter.
5. Put a muffin pan upside down and assemble the taco chaffle upon the cups to make into a taco shell. Put aside for a few minutes.
6. When it is firm, fill it with your favorite Taco Meat fillings. Serve.

Enjoy this delicious keto crispy taco chaffle shell with your favorite toppings.

Chapter 3- Keto Cakes and Cupcakes

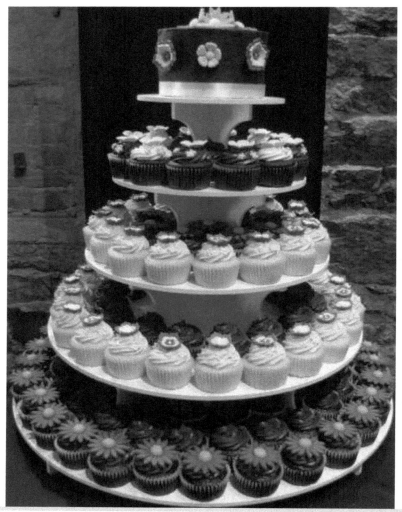

1. Chocolate Cake with Chocolate Icing

Prep. Time: 10 minutes

Cook Time: 25 minutes

Servings: 9 slices

The serving size is 1 slice

Nutrition as per serving:

358kcal / 33g fat / 11g carbs / 6g fiber / 8g protein = 5g net carbs

Ingredients

- Coconut flour 3/4 cup
- Granular sweetener 3/4 cup
- Cocoa powder 1/2 cup
- Baking powder 2tsps

- Eggs 6
- Heavy whipping cream 2/3 cup
- Melted butter 1/2 cup
- For chocolate icing
- Heavy whipping cream 1 cup
- Keto granular sweetener 1/4 cup
- Vanilla extracts 1tsp.
- Cocoa powder sifted 1/3 cup

Directions

1. Heat the oven up to 350F.
2. Oil a cake pan of 8x8.
3. In a large mixing bowl, put all the cake ingredients to blend well with an electric mixer or a stand mixer.
4. Transfer the batter to the oiled pan and put in the heated oven for 25 minutes or till a toothpick inserted in the center comes out clean.
5. Take out from the oven. Leave to cool fully before icing.
6. Prepare the Icing
7. With an electric mixer, beat the whipping cream until stiff peaks form. Include the cocoa powder, swerve, and vanilla. Keep beating until just combined.
8. Spread the icing evenly all over the cake and serve. Keep any remains in the refrigerator.

2. 4 Ingredients Cheesecake Fluff

Prep. Time: 10 minutes

Servings: 6

The serving size is ½ cup

Nutrition as per serving:

258kcal / 27g fat / 4g carbs / 0g fiber / 4g protein = 4g net carbs

Ingredients

- Heavy Whipping Cream1 Cup
- Cream Cheese, Softened 1 Brick (8 oz.)
- Lemon Zest 1 tsp.
- Keto-friendly Granular Sweetener 1/2 Cup

Directions

1. Prepare the Fluff
2. Put the heavy cream in a bowl of a stand mixer and beat until stiff peaks begin to form. An electric beater or a hand beater can also be used.
3. Transfer the whipped cream into a separate bowl and put aside
4. To the same stand mixer bowl, add the cream cheese (softened), sweetener, zest, and whisk until smooth.

5. Now add the whipped cream to the cream cheese into the mixer bowl. Fold with a spatula gently till it is halfway combined. Finish whipping with the stand mixer until smooth.
6. Top with your fave toppings and serve.

3. Mug Cake Peanut Butter, Chocolate or Vanilla

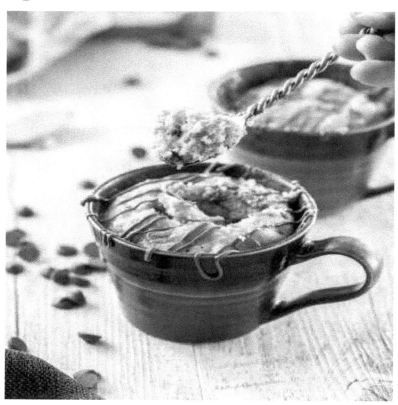

Prep. Time: 4 minutes

Cook Time: 1 minute

Servings: 1

The serving size is 1 mug cake

Nutrition as per serving:

(For mug cake with almond flour: chocolate flavor and no chocolate chips)

312 kcal / 7 carbs/ 28g fat / 12g protein/4g fiber = 3 net carbs

(Peanut butter flavor and no chocolate chips)

395 kcal / 8 carbs /35g fat / 15g protein/4g fiber = 5 net carb

(Vanilla flavor and no chocolate chips)

303 kcal / 5 carbs/ 28g fat / 11g protein /2g fiber = 3 net carb

Ingredients

- Butter melted 1 Tbsp.
- Almond flour 3 Tbsp. or Coconut flour 1 Tbsp.

- Granular Sweetener 2 Tbsp.
- Sugar-free Peanut butter 1 Tbsp. (For Peanut Butter flavor)
- Cocoa powder 1 Tbsp. (For Chocolate flavor)
- Baking powder ½ tsp.
- Egg, beaten 1
- Sugar-free Chocolate Chips 1 Tbsp.
- Vanilla few drops

Directions

For Vanilla flavor

1. In a microwave-proof coffee mug, heat the butter for 10 seconds to melt in the microwave.
2. Include the almond flour or coconut flour, baking powder, sweetener, beaten egg and vanilla. Combine well.
3. For 60 seconds, microwave on high, ensuring not to overcook; otherwise, it will come out dry. Sprinkle keto chocolate chips on top if preferred or stir in before cooking.

For Chocolate flavor

In a microwave-proof coffee mug, heat the butter for 10 seconds to melt in the microwave. Include the almond flour or coconut flour, cocoa powder, sweetener, baking powder, beaten egg and vanilla. Combine well. For 60 seconds, microwave on high, ensuring not to overcook; it will come out dry. Sprinkle keto chocolate chips on top if preferred.

For Peanut Butter flavor

1. In a microwave-proof coffee mug, heat the butter for 10 seconds to melt in the microwave.
2. Include the almond flour or coconut flour, baking powder, sweetener, beaten egg and vanilla. Combine well. Stir in peanut butter. For 60 seconds, microwave on high, ensuring not to overcook; otherwise, it will come out dry. Sprinkle keto chocolate chips on top if preferred.

Directions for Baking: Bake in an oven-safe small bowl. Bake in the oven for 15 to 20 minutes at 350.

4. Chocolate Coconut Flour Cupcakes

Prep. Time: 10 minutes

Cook Time: 25 minutes

Servings: 12 cupcakes

The serving size is 1 cupcake

Nutrition as per serving:

268 kcal / 22g fat / 6g carbs / 3g fiber / 6g protein = 3g net carbs

Ingredients

For Cupcakes:

- Butter melted 1/2 cup
- Cocoa powder 7 tbsp.
- Instant coffee granules 1 tsp (optional)
- Eggs at room temperature 7
- Vanilla extracts 1 tsp
- Coconut flour 2/3 cup
- Baking powder 2 tsp
- Swerve sweetener 2/3 cup
- Salt 1/2 tsp
- Hemp milk or unsweetened almond milk 1/2 cup (+more)

For Espresso Buttercream:

- Hot water 2 tbsp.
- Instant coffee or instant espresso powder 2 tsp
- Whipping cream 1/2 cup
- Butter softened 6 tbsp.
- Cream cheese softened 4 oz.
- Swerve powdered sweetener 1/2 cup

Directions

For Cupcakes:

1. Heat the oven up to 350F and line silicone liners or parchment on a muffin tin.
2. Mix together the cocoa powder, melted butter, and espresso powder in a large mixing bowl,
3. Include the vanilla and eggs and whisk until well combined. Now add in the coconut flour, baking powder, salt and sweetener, and mix until smooth.
4. Pour the almond milk in and stir. If the batter is very thick, add in 1 tbsp. of almond milk at a time to thin it out. It should not be pourable but of scoopable consistency.
5. Scoop the batter equally among the prepared muffin tins and put in the oven's center rack, baking for 20-25 minutes. Check the cupcakes with a tester inserted into the center comes out clean, then cupcakes are done. Leave to cool in the pan for 5 to 10 minutes, and then cool completely on a wire rack.

For Buttercream:

1. Dissolve the coffee in hot water. Put aside.
2. Whip cream using an electric mixer until stiff peaks are formed. Put aside.
3. Beat cream cheese, butter, and sweetener all together in a medium mixing bowl until creamy. Include coffee mixture and mix until combined. fold in the whipped cream Using a rubber spatula carefully till well combined.
4. Layer frosting on the cooled cupcakes with an offset spatula or a knife.

5. Low-carb red velvet cupcakes/ cake

Prep. Time: 15-30 minutes

Cook Time: 20-25 minutes

Servings: 12 slice

The serving size is 1 slice

Nutrition as per serving:

193kcals / 12g fat / 6.4g carbs / 1g fiber / 5.9g protein = 5.4g net carbs

Ingredients

- Almond flour 1+ 3/4 cups
- Swerve confectioner sweetener (not substitutes) 2/3 cup
- Cocoa powder 2 tbsp.
- Baking powder 2tsp.
- Baking soda 1/2tsp.
- Eggs 2
- Full fat coconut milk 1/2 cup + 2 tbsp.
- Olive oil 3 tbsp.
- Apple cider vinegar 1 tbsp.
- Vanilla extract 1 tbsp.
- Red food coloring 2 tbsp.

For frosting

- Cream cheese at room temperature 1 container (8 oz.)
- Butter softened 2 ½ tbsp.
- Swerve confectioner sweetener 1 cup
- Coconut milk 2 ½ tbsp.
- Vanilla extract 1tsp.
- Salt 1/8tsp.

**Double Frosting for Layer Cake

Directions

1. Preheat oven to 350 degrees
2. In a large mixing bowl, add the wet ingredients, eggs, milk, vanilla extract, olive oil, apple cider vinegar and food coloring. Blend until smooth.
3. Now sift together the cocoa powder, Swerve Confectioner, baking powder and baking soda, add to the wet ingredients, and incorporate it into the batter with an electric mixer or a hand whisk.
4. Lastly, sift in the almond flour. Moving the flour back and forth with a whisk will speed up the process significantly. Fold the sifted flour gently into the batter till smooth and all is well incorporated. Use the batter immediately.
5. To make Cupcakes: Scoop batter into the muffin liners, fill only up to 2/3 of liner -do not over-fill. Ensure the oven is heated, put in the oven for 15 minutes at 350 degrees, and then turn the muffin tin in 180 degrees and cook for an extra 10 minutes. (Bear in mind, oven times vary occasionally - humidity and altitude can impact things, so watch closely as they may need a few minutes more or even less).
6. Take out from the oven, do not remove from pan and set aside to cool completely.
7. For Layer Cake: 2 Layer- line parchment paper in two cake pans (8 inches each) and oil the sides. Transfer batter to both pans evenly. Use a wet spatula to spread the batter

smoothly. Apply the same process for three layers, but using thinner pans as dividing the batter three ways-every layers will become thin.

8. Place pans into oven for 20-25 minutes baking at 350 degrees. Cautiously turn the pans 180 degrees halfway through baking and cover lightly with a foil. At 20 to 25 minutes, take out the pans; they will be a bit soft. Set them aside to cool completely. When they are cool, take a knife and run it around the side of the pan and turn them over carefully onto a plate or cooling rack and leave them for an extra 5 to 10 minutes before icing.

9. Meanwhile, prepare. Blend the softened butter and cream cheese together With an electric beater. Include milk and vanilla extract and beat again. Lastly, sift in the Swerve, salt mixing well one last time. If you want a thicker frosting, chill it in the refrigerator. Or adding more Swerve will give a thicker texture or add more milk to make it thinner. * For a layer cake, double the frosting recipe.

10. Spread or pipe frosting onto cupcakes, sprinkle some decoration if desired and enjoy!! To frost layer cake, it is simpler to first chill the layers in the freezer. Then frost and pile each layer to end frost the sides and top.

Keep any leftovers in a sealed box and refrigerate. Enjoy!

6. Vanilla Cupcakes

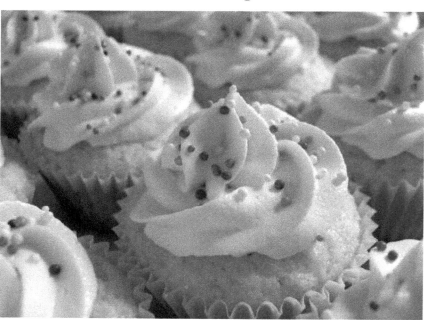

Prep. Time: 5 minutes

Cook Time: 20 minutes

Servings: 10 Cupcakes

The serving size is 1 cupcake

Nutrition as per serving:

153kcal / 13g fat / 4g carbs / 2g fiber / 5g protein = 2g net carbs

Ingredients

- Butter 1/2 cup
- Keto granulated sweetener 2/3 cup
- Vanilla extract 2 tsp
- Eggs whisked * See notes 6 large
- Milk of choice ** See notes 2 tbsp.
- Coconut flour 1/2 cup
- Baking powder 1 tsp
- Keto vanilla frosting 1 batch

Directions

1. Heat the oven up to 350F/180C. Place muffin liners in a 12-cup muffin tin and oil 10 of them.
2. Beat the butter, salt, sugar, eggs and vanilla extract together in a big mixing bowl when combined-well include the milk and mix until blended.
3. In another bowl, sift the baking powder and coconut flour together. Add the wet ingredients to the dry and mix until combined.
4. Pour the batter equally into the ten muffin cups, filling up to ¾ full. Place the cupcakes on the middle rack and bake for 17 to 20 minutes until the muffin top springs back to touch
5. Remove the muffin pan from the oven, set it aside to cool for 10 minutes, and then cool completely on a wire rack. Frost, when cooled.

7. Healthy Flourless Fudge Brownies

Prep. Time: 5 minutes

Cook Time: 20 minutes

Servings: 12 servings

The serving size is 1 Brownie

Nutrition as per serving:

86kcal / 5g fat / 5g carbs / 3g fiber / 7g protein = 2g net carbs

Ingredients

- Pumpkin puree 2 cups
- Almond butter 1 cup
- Cocoa powder 1/2 cup
- Granulated sweetener (or liquid stevia drops) 1/4 cup

For the Chocolate Coconut Frosting

- Chocolate chips 2 cups
- Coconut milk canned 1 cup
- For the chocolate protein frosting
- Protein powder, chocolate flavor 2 scoops
- Granulated sweetener 1-2 tbsp.

- Seed or nut butter of choice 1-2 tbsp.
- Milk or liquid *1 tbsp.

For the Cheese Cream Frosting

- Cream cheese 125 grams
- Cocoa powder 1-2 tbsp.
- Granulated sweetener of choice 1-2 tbsp.

Directions

1. For the fudge brownies
2. Heat the oven up to 350 degrees, oil a loaf pan or small cake pan and put aside.
3. Melt the nut butter in a small microwave-proof bowl. In a big mixing bowl, put in the pumpkin puree, dark cocoa powder, nut butter, and combine very well.
4. Transfer the mixture to the oiled pan and put in preheated oven for around 20 to 25 minutes or until fully baked. Remove from the oven, set aside to cool completely. When cooled, apply the frosting and chill for about 30 minutes to settle.

Preparing the cream cheese or protein frosting:

1. In a big mixing bowl, mix together all the ingredients and beat well. With a tablespoon. keep adding dairy-free milk till a frosting consistency is reached.
2. For the coconut chocolate ganache
3. In a microwave-proof bowl, combine all the ingredients and heat gradually until just mixed- whisk till a glossy and thick frosting remains.

8. Healthy Keto Chocolate Raspberry Mug Cake

Prep. Time: 1 minute

Cook Time: 1 minute

Servings: 1 serving

The serving size is 1 mug cake

Nutrition as per serving:

152kcal / 8g fat / 13g carbs / 8g fiber / 7g protein = 5g net carbs

Ingredients

- Coconut flour 1 tbsp.
- Granulated sweetener of choice 1 tbsp.
- Cocoa powder 2 tbsp.
- Baking powder 1/4 tsp
- Sunflower seed butter (or any seed or nut butter) 1 tbsp.
- Pumpkin puree 3 tbsp.
- Frozen or fresh raspberries 1/4 cup
- Coconut milk unsweetened 1-2 tbsp.

Directions

1. In a microwave-proof mug, put in the dry ingredients and stir well.

2. Add in the rest of the ingredients, except for milk and raspberries, and combine until a thick batter is formed.
3. Stir in the raspberries and add one tbsp. of milk. Add extra milk if the batter gets too thick. Place in microwave and cook for 1 to 2 minutes. Should come out gooey in the center. If you overcook, it will become dry.

Oven Directions

1. Heat oven up to 180C.
2. Oil an oven-proof ramekin. Add the prepared batter and put in the oven for 10-12 minutes, or until done.

9. Keto Avocado Brownies

Prep. Time: 10 minutes

Cook Time: 30 minutes

Servings: 12 squares

Nutrition as per serving:

155kcal / 14g fat / 13g carbs / 10g fiber / 4g protein = 2.8g net carbs

Ingredients

- Avocado, mashed 1 cup
- Vanilla 1/2 tsp
- Cocoa powder 4 tbsp.
- Refined coconut oil (or ghee, butter, lard, shortening) 3 tbsp.
- Eggs 2
- Lily's chocolate chips melted 1/2 cup (100 g)

Dry Ingredients

- Blanched almond flour 3/4 cup
- Baking soda 1/4 tsp
- Baking powder 1 tsp
- Salt 1/4 tsp
- Erythritol 1/4 cup (see sweetener note *1)
- Stevia powder 1 tsp (see sweetener note *1)

Directions

1. Heat the oven up to 350F/ 180C.
2. Sift together the dry ingredients in a small bowl and stir.
3. Place the Peeled avocados in a food processor and process until smooth.
4. One by one, add all the wet ingredients into the food processor, processing every few seconds
5. Now include the dry ingredients into the food processor and blend until combined.
6. Line a parchment paper in a baking dish (of 12"x8") and transfer the batter into it. Spread evenly and put in the heated oven. Cook for 30 minutes or the center springs back to touch. It should be soft to touch.
7. Remove from oven, set aside to cool fully before cutting into 12 slices.

10. Low Carb-1 minute Cinnamon Roll Mug Cake

Prep. Time: 1 minute

Cook Time: 1 minute

Servings: 1 serving

The serving size is 1mug

Nutrition as per serving:

132kcal / 4g fat / 6g carbs / 2g fiber / 25g protein = 4g net carbs

Ingredients

- Protein powder, vanilla flavor 1 scoop
- Baking powder 1/2 tsp
- Coconut flour 1 tbsp.
- Cinnamon 1/2 tsp
- Granulated sweetener 1 tbsp.
- Egg 1 large
- Almond milk, unsweetened 1/4 cup
- Vanilla extract 1/4 tsp
- Granulated sweetener 1 tsp
- Cinnamon 1/2 tsp

For the glaze

- Coconut butter melted 1 tbsp.
- Almond milk 1/2 tsp
- Cinnamon a pinch

Directions

1. Oil a microwave-proof mug. In a small bowl, add the protein powder, coconut flour, baking powder, sweetener, cinnamon and mix well.
2. Add in the egg and stir into the flour mixture. Include the vanilla extract and milk. If the batter is too dry, keep adding milk until a thick consistency is reached.
3. Pour this batter into the oiled mug. Sprinkle extra cinnamon and keto granulated sweetener over the top and swirl. Place in microwave and cook for 60 seconds, or till the center is just cooked. Do not overcook, or it will come out dry. Drizzle the glaze on top and enjoy!
4. Prepare glaze by mixing all ingredients and use.

11. Double Chocolate Muffins

Prep. Time: 10 minutes

Cook Time: 15 minutes

Servings: 12 muffins

The serving size is 1 muffin

Nutrition as per serving:

280 kcal / 27g fat / 7g carbs / 4g fiber / 7g protein = 3g net carbs

Ingredients

- Almond flour 2 cup
- Cocoa powder unsweetened 3/4 cup
- Swerve sweetener 1/4 cup
- Baking powder 1 1/2 tsp.
- Kosher salt 1 tsp.
- Butter melted 1 cup (2 sticks)
- Eggs 3 large
- Pure vanilla extract 1 tsp.
- Dark chocolate chips, sugar-free (like lily's) 1 cup

Directions

1. Heat oven up to 350° and line cupcake liners in a muffin tin. In a big bowl, stir together almond flour, Swerve, cocoa powder, salt and baking powder. Include eggs, melted butter and vanilla and mix until combined.
2. Stir in the chocolate chips.
3. Pour batter equally in muffin cups and bake for 12 minutes or until the muffin top springs back to touch.

Chapter 4- Keto Fat Bombs

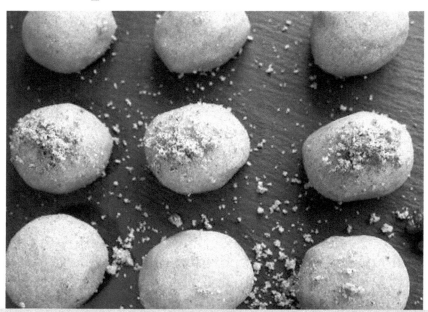

1. Cheesecake Fat Bombs

Prep. Time: 5 minutes

Servings: 24Fat Bombs

The serving size is 1 Fat Bomb

Nutrition as per serving:

108kcal / 12g fat / 1g carbs / 1g fiber / 1g protein = 0g net carbs

Ingredients

- Heavy Cream 4 oz.
- Cream cheese at room temperature 8 oz.
- Erythritol 2-3 tbsp.
- Coconut oil or butter 4 oz.
- Vanilla extracts 2tsp.
- Baking chocolate or coconut for decorating

Directions

1. In a big mixing bowl, add all the ingredients and mix for 1-2 minutes with an electric mixer until well combined and creamy.
2. Spoon mixture into an unlined or lined mini cupcake tin. Chill for 1-2 hours in the refrigerator or freezer for about 30 minutes.
3. Take out from the cupcake tins and store them in a sealed container. It can be refrigerated for up to two weeks.

2. Brownie Fat Bombs

Prep. Time: 15 minutes

Servings: 16 fat bombs

The serving size is 2 fat bombs

Nutrition as per serving:

174 kcal / 16g fat / 4g carbs / 2g fiber / 3g protein = 2g net carbs

Ingredients

- Ghee 1/4 cup
- Cocoa butter 1 oz.
- Vanilla extract 1/2 tsp
- Salt 1/4 tsp
- Raw cacao powder 6 tbsp.
- Swerve Sweetener powdered 1/3 cup
- Water 2 tbsp.
- Almond butter 1/3 cup
- Nuts, chopped (optional) 1/4 cup

Directions

1. melt the cocoa butter and ghee together In a heat-safe bowl placed over a pot of simmering water,
2. Add in the sweetener, cacao powder, salt and vanilla extract. This mixture will be smooth and thin.
3. Stir in the water and beat the mixture till it thickens to the consistency of a thick frosting.
4. Mix in the nut butter with a rubber spatula. The mixture will look like cookie dough. Mix in the coarsely chopped nuts.
5. Shape into 1 inch sized balls (will make about 16) and chill until firm.

3. Coffee Fat Bombs

Prep. Time: 10 minutes

Servings: 8 Fat Bombs

The serving size is 1 Fat Bomb

Nutrition as per serving:

140 kcal / 14g fat / 4g carbs / 2g fiber / 1.5g protein = 2g net carbs

Ingredients

- Cream Cheese, Full-fat 8 Oz.
- Butter Unsalted, ½ cup (1 Stick)
- Instant Coffee 1 to 2 Tbsps.

- Chocolate Chips, Low Carb, heaped ¼ Cup
- Confectioners Erythritol heaped ⅓ Cup
- Cocoa Powder, Unsweetened 1½ Tbsp.

Directions

1. In a large bowl, place the butter and cream cheese (both should be at room temperature)
2. Combine them with an electric mixer until smooth.
3. Then include all the remaining ingredients in the bowl, blending until well-combined
4. Scoop out the batter with a tablespoon or a cookie scoop to make around 12 bombs. Place them on a baking sheet lined with parchment. Chill for about 3 hours.

4. Peanut Butter Fat Bombs

Prep. Time: 10 minutes

Servings: 12 fat bombs

The serving size is 1/2 fat bomb

Nutrition as per serving:

247 kcal / 24.3g fat / 3.2g carbs / 1.2g fiber / 3.6g protein = 2g net carbs

Ingredients

For fat bomb

- Natural peanut butter (no sugar) 3/4 cup
- Coconut oil (melted) 1/2 cup
- Vanilla extract 1 tsp.
- Liquid stevia 3 – 4 drops
- Sea salt 1/4 tsp.

For Ganache

- Coconut oil 6 tbsp.
- Cocoa powder 1 tbsp.
- Liquid stevia 1 – 2 drops

Directions

1. Mix the peanut butter, coconut oil, vanilla extract, salt, and liquid stevia together in a small mixing bowl, beat until creamy and smooth.
2. Line muffin paper cups in a six-cup-muffin tray. Fill each cup with about 3 tbsp. of the peanut butter mixture.
3. Refrigerate for about 1 hour to solidify.
4. Meanwhile, beat together the ingredients for Ganache until it's silky.
5. Drizzle about one tbsp. of the chocolate ganache on every fat bomb.
6. Chill for about 30 minutes and enjoy.

5. Cream Cheese Pumpkin Spiced Fat Bombs

Prep. Time: 10 minutes

Servings: 12 Fat Bombs

The serving size is 1 Fat Bomb

Nutrition as per serving:

80 kcal / 7.5g fat / 2g carbs / 0.25g fiber / 1.5g protein = 1.75g net carbs

Ingredients

- Pure pumpkin ⅔ cup
- Pumpkin pie spice ½ tsp
- Cream cheese, full-fat 8 oz.
- Butter melted 3 tbsps.
- Confectioner's erythritol 3 tbsps.

Directions

1. Place all the ingredients in a large bowl and mix with an electric mixer until combined.
2. Make 12 equal-sized balls from the dough. Place paper liners in a mini-muffin tin and place the PB cookie dough in the muffin tin.
3. Chill for a minimum of 2 hours

Note:

If the pumpkin pie spice is not available, make some with the following ingredients

¼ tsp cinnamon, a pinch of (each) - nutmeg, cloves, ginger and allspice.

6. Brownie Truffles

Prep. Time: 5 minutes

Cook Time: 5 minutes

Servings: 20 Truffles

The serving size is 1 Truffle

Nutrition as per serving:

97kcal / 8g fat / 5g carbs / 3g fiber / 4g protein = 2g net carbs

Ingredients

- Sticky sweetener, keto-friendly 1/2 cup of choice
- Homemade Nutella 2 cups
- Coconut flour 3/4 cup (or almond flour 1 ½ cup)
- Chocolate chips, sugar-free 2 cups

Directions

1. Combine the coconut/almond flour, sticky sweetener and chocolate spread in a big mixing bowl. Add a bit more syrup or liquid; if the mixture is too thick, it should become a creamy dough.
2. Place parchment paper on a large plate. Shape into small balls with your hands, and set on the plate. Chill.

3. Melt the sugar-free chocolate chips. Take the truffles from the refrigerator. Immediately, coat each truffle with the melted chocolate, making sure all are evenly coated.
4. Set back on the lined
5. Plate and chill until firm.

7. Coconut Strawberry Fat Bombs

Prep. Time: 10 minutes

Servings: 20 fat bombs

The serving size is 1fat Bomb

Nutrition as per serving:

132kcals / 14.3g fat / 0.9g carbs / 0g fiber / 0.4g protein = 0.9g net carbs

Ingredients

For Coconut base:

- Coconut cream 1 1/2 cups
- Coconut oil (melted) 1/2 cup
- Stevia liquid 1/2 tsp.
- Lime juice 1 tbsp.

For Strawberry topping:

- Fresh chopped strawberries 2 oz.
- Coconut oil (melted) 1/2 cup
- Liquid stevia 5 – 8 drops

Directions

Prepare the coconut base:

1. In a high-speed blender, place all the coconut base ingredients and blend them completely until combined and smooth.
2. Distribute the mixture evenly into an ice cube tray, muffin tray, or a candy mold, leaving room for the topping.
3. Chill in the freezer to set for about 20 minutes.

For the Strawberry topping:

1. In a blender, put all the ingredients for the strawberry topping, then blend until smooth.
2. When the base is set, spoon the strawberry mixture equally over each one.
3. Refrigerate the fat bombs for about 2 hours and enjoy.

8. Raspberry & White Chocolate Fat Bombs

Prep. Time: 5 minutes

Servings: 10-12 fat bombs

The serving size is 1 fat Bomb

Nutrition as per serving:

153kcal / 16g fat / 1.5g carbs / 0.4g fiber / 0.2g protein = 1.2g net carbs

Ingredients

- Cacao butter 2 oz.
- Coconut oil 1/2 cup
- Raspberries freeze-dried 1/2 cup
- Erythritol sweetener, powdered (like swerve) 1/4 cup

Directions

1. Place paper liners in a 12-cup muffin pan.
2. In a small pot, heat the cacao butter and coconut oil on low flame until melted completely. Take off the pot from heat.
3. Blend the freeze-dried raspberries in a blender or food processor, or coffee grinder.
4. Include the sweetener and powdered berries into the pot, stirring to dissolve the sweetener.
5. Distribute the mixture evenly between the muffin cups. Don't worry if the raspberry powder sinks to the bottom. Just stir the mixture when pouring them into each mold to distribute the raspberry powder in each mold.
6. Chill until hard. Enjoy.

9. Almond Joy Fat Bombs (3 Ingredients)

Prep. Time: 2 minutes

Cook Time: 3 minutes

Servings: 24 cups

The serving size is 1 cup

Nutrition as per serving:

72kcal / 8g fat / 6g carbs / 4g fiber / 2g protein = 2g net carbs

Ingredients

- Coconut butter softened 1/4 cup
- Chocolate chips, sugar-free, divided 20 oz.
- Almonds 24 whole

Directions

1. Place muffin liners in a 24-cup mini muffin tin and put them aside.
2. Melt 3/4 of the sugar-free chocolate chips in a microwave-proof bowl. Distribute the chocolate mixture equally into all the muffin liners. Also, scrape down all the chocolate coated on the sides. Chill until firm.

3. When the chocolate is hard, spoon in the melted coconut butter evenly into every chocolate cup, leaving room for chocolate filling on top. Add in more softened coconut butter if needed.
4. Melt the rest of the chocolate chips and with it, cover each of the chocolate coconut cups. Place an almond on top of each cup and chill until firm.

10. Pecan pie fat bombs

Prep. Time: 15 minutes

Servings: 18 balls

The serving size is 2 balls

Nutrition as per serving

121 kcal / 12g fat / 3.8g carbs / 2.9g fiber / 2g protein = 0.9g net carbs

Ingredients

- Pecans, (or any nut) 1½ cup s
- Coconut butter, ¼ cup
- Coconut shredded ½ cup
- Chia seeds 2 tbsp.
- Pecan butter (or any nut butter) 2 tbsp.
- Flax meal 2 tbsp.
- Coconut oil 1tsp.
- Hemp seeds 2 tbsp.
- Vanilla extract ½tsp.
- Cinnamon 1½tsp.
- Kosher salt ¼tsp.

Directions

1. Add the ingredients altogether in a food processor. Process for a minute or two to break down the mixture. First, it will become powdery. Then it will stick together but remain crumbly.
2. Continue to process until the oils begin to expel a bit, and the mixture will begin to stick together easily –be cautious not to process excessively, or you will have nut butter.
3. Using a tablespoon or small cookie scooper, scoop to make equal pieces of the mixture. Roll them into balls with your hands placing them all on a large plate. Chill for about 30 mins.
4. Keep in a sealed container or a zip-lock bag in the freezer or refrigerator.

11. PB. Cookie Dough Fat Bomb

Prep. Time: 10 minutes

Servings: 12 Fat Bombs

The serving size is 1 Fat Bomb

Nutrition as per serving:

135kcal / 11g fat / 5g carbs / 3.5g fiber / 4g protein = 1.5g net carbs

Ingredients

- Lily's chocolate chips ⅓ cup
- Almond flour, superfine 1 cup
- Natural peanut butter 6 tbsps.
- Confectioner's erythritol 2 tbsps.
- Coconut oil (melted) 1 tbsps.
- Vanilla extract 1 tsp
- Salt, a pinch

Directions

1. Place all the ingredients in a large bowl and mix with a spoon until crumbly.
2. Form a dough ball with your hands.
3. Line parchment paper on a baking sheet. Scoop out equal-sized 12 cookie dough fat bombs.
4. Chill for about an hour
5. Once they are done setting, keep in a sealed bag in the fridge.

Conclusion

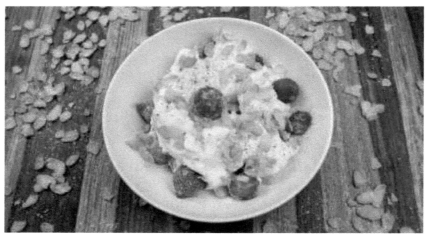

When going on a ketogenic diet, one retains modest protein consumption but increases their fat intake. The transition to a low-carb diet brings your body into a ketosis state, where fat is used for energy compared to carbohydrates.

It takes some time for fats to decompose through the digestive tract and delay the decomposition of the carbohydrates into sugar, maintain our blood sugar concentrations steady and allow us to feel satiated longer. Based on observational evidence, incorporating a tablespoonful of coconut oil into your diet every day may also result in lower weight.

You may also need to monitor the portion sizes, but as fat is intrinsically pleasing, having one for breakfast will help deter eating during meals.

When consuming high-fat meals, including keto fat bombs, you will further encourage weight reduction by decreasing appetite for the next meal. Be it fat bombs or cheesy waffles or any other hi fat low-carb dessert, they are a dieter's dream come true.

Following the keto diet can positively impact one's brain function.

Advantages of the ketogenic diet and fat bombs.

Keto fat bombs may be seen as a way to reduce sugar habits.

Ketogenic fat bombs are simple to produce, easy to keep, and easy to eat; they often need fewer ingredients than other foods.

Ketogenic fat bombs are tasty and have a broad variety of low-carb recipes.

Ketogenic fat bombs are quick to produce, are easy to store, and are ready to consume at any time.

In this book, you will find the best and easy to prepare keto cakes, chaffles, and yummy high-fat recipes that will fulfill your cravings for desserts after meals or snacks when you don't feel too hungry. Enjoy these recipes by yourself, or even better, share the joy with family and friends!

CPSIA information can be obtained
at www.ICGtesting.com
Printed in the USA
BVHW091338220321
603174BV00014B/323